How I Cured My Cancer In 4 Months

Λ truc story of a woman's battle
with cancer and her ultimate rapid cure

Rosemarie Scarpignato

DISCLAIMER

The author and publishers are not responsible for the results of any actions taken on the basis of information in this publication. All information contained in this book is anecdotal only and if other medical advice is required, people should consult their health professionals before embarking on any treatments.

Foreword

As I write this book I ask myself am I qualified to write such a book, and the answer is a resounding "YES". Although I've had no formal medical training, I have read extensively many books on Cancer cures, articles on health, and I have really delved into the rudiments of foods; what are healthy foods and what are not. I have also attended many Seminars over the years, conducted by many Health Professionals, where I learned eating healthily can put the brakes on illness of all kinds including cancer.

My journey into Natural Health came about when I turned 35 and suddenly developed Rheumatoid Arthritis, which was brought on by a car accident. I received a whiplash from the accident and I was never the same after that. The shock of the car accident brought on an auto-immune response, which lowers the body's immune system where the body attacks itself, hence Rheumatoid Arthritis became my constant companion. My hands and feet were swollen and very painful, something I had never experienced before.

The Medical Profession had no answers for me, as I started taking anti-inflammatories, which seemed to work for a while; I even changed medications a couple of times, but later on I became immune to them and they only upset my stomach, so I discontinued using them.

Finally a friend suggested I consult a naturopath whom she worked for, so I went and had a long consultation with him. During the consultation he went over my diet thoroughly and noticed I had a lot of inflammation and found that my body was very acidic, due to the very acidic diet I was on. The main culprits were too much meat, wheat and dairy foods and not enough fruits and vegetables, especially raw. Whilst speaking to the naturopath I learned about which foods are acidic to the body and which foods are alkaline (most fruits and vegetables). I think people today are eating the standard western diet, which is obviously causing cancer and other diseases, so rife in western civilisation.

The reason I have written this book is to convey the message to readers is that cancer doesn't have to be a death sentence. Even in its advanced stages, cancer can be stopped in its tracks, by using a plant-based, semi-vegetarian and detoxifying diet. I am a testimony to my own cancer story where I was diagnosed with Non-Hodgkins Lymphoma and Stage 2 Bone Cancer which was at an advanced stage. I decided I was going to cure myself and I did achieve that goal in just four short months.

I will be happy if this book can make people aware that they too can heal their bodies from illness naturally and with a minimum of pharmaceutical drugs.

Acknowledgements

I would like to thank several people during the writing of this book.

First and foremost, a big thank you to my wonderful husband, Joe who took over many of the household duties, such as shopping, food preparation etc. as I was on the finishing stages of the book.

To my loving children, Tommy and Melissa who kept encouraging me to keep writing my story, even though it was a bit tedious at times.

I want to thank the following people for information on my early ancestry. They are as follows: My beloved Aunt Jessie Sidoti, our Matriarch, who is now in her mid-nineties, and cousins, Sylvie Mullens, Rosie Rocca, Neil Arena, Christine Hoole, Sebastian Anthony Arena, Sebastian Leo Arena, and Josie Franckin.

I want to thank my daughter-in-law, Charryse, who, with her technical computer expertise, AND patience assisted me on the many occasions when I had computer issues.

I would also like to thank Mary Jarrett, Sales Executive of Griffin Press for her assistance and recommending David Bradbury.

David Bradbury is the typesetter who helped assist me prepare my files, and I want to give him a big thank you for his invaluable advice in the many aspects of assisting me through the publishing process.

Niki Palmer, Bestselling Amazon Co-author creates books to assist parents and children with health, and social issues is delighted to have the opportunity to assist me with my book on healing cancer the natural way. Niki's books can be found at www. westminsterdesigns.com.au.

Photography on the covers of this book are from Simon Carroll, who is the owner of "Living image Photography" a professional portrait studio based in Richmond Victoria, who has a team of gifted individuals who all specialise in their true love and passion – creating natural portraits of children, dogs and their families and transforming their images into beautiful finished artwork.

Contents

Chapter 1

In The Beginning

Cancer! The very word fills terror in the mind and hearts of all people. What is this dreaded disease that is killing thousands of people every day all over the world. How did we get to this point? It is now 1 in 2 people that are afflicted with Cancer in Western Countries. In 2011 in the United States alone, over 500,000 people died from cancer. In Australia the staggering statistics read like this: 2600 women die from breast cancer annually, 3300 men die annually from prostate cancer, 4000 people die annually from bowel cancer, 1200 people die annually from brain cancer, 800 women die annually from ovarian cancer, 1200 people die annually from brain cancer and leukaemia is also killing over 20,000 people each year, and the list goes on. There is not enough room on this page to list the statistics of all the cancers. In order to try and work out how we got to these astounding statistics let us go father back to the beginning.

Let Medicine Be Thy Food

According to Wikipedia, Hippocrates, the Father of Modern Medicine, was made famous by the often repeated quotation" Let food be thy medicine and medicine be thy food" and was an ancient Greek physician of the Age of Pericles, who was born in 460BC.

He believed that disease was caused naturally by diet and living habits and environmental factors. Born ahead of his time he was considered one of the most notable figures of western medicine, and during his time as a physician treated illness with fasting and only eating healthy foods, without harmful drugs. It is believed he himself lived to a ripe old age, the correct age is not exactly known, probably his late eighties, by practising the diet and lifestyle he recommended to his patients.

In Biblical Times
Old Age Was Common

In Biblical times, Moses, along with his contemporaries many of whom were centenarians, lived to be about 120; (so it is written) old age was common, not like today where old age is rare. It must've been their diets which comprised fruits and vegetables which didn't have chemicals sprayed on them. They ate the foods that nature intended them to eat from God's great garden. They ate foods like unleavened bread, natural cheese; they rarely ate meat, and fattened a calf for consumption only on very special occasions, they also ate pulses, and drank pure water which had no harmful chemicals in it, unlike today. Perhaps this killer disease, cancer is a punishment to society for rejecting the pure natural foods provided that nature intended them to eat, instead giving in to all the trendy, modern poisonous foods so prevalent in today's society. The deadly diseases they encountered in those times were mainly leprosy, which was highly contagious and many people eventually died from it and consumption, or better known today as TB which killed many people in those times. Looking at pictures in the Bible I notice that men in biblical times had long thick hair; could it be the naturally healthy diet, (free from chemicals) that they ate in those times, not like today's times in western society where so many men are going bald younger and younger?

The average life expectancy for the US male is 80yrs and females is 75, Australian males 83yrs and females is 79, with the UK similar averages; although many people are dying much younger than that including children and babies, but we will deal with that in a later chapter.

The Longest Living Peoples Of The World

According to knowledgeable Australian Health Educator, Roger French, and author of the book "The man who lived in three centuries" writes "Where do people get the idea that we're over the hill at 40? Today the goalposts have shifted and there's a new catchphrase about ageing: 50 is what 40 used to be. However, the slide towards degenerative disease and premature ageing is still very common after 40 to 50 really good years. We have only to look at primitive peoples – plus some modern day examples – to see just what lifespan we are capable of and how brilliantly well designed the human body really is. Primitive peoples that were studied before Western influence got to them include the Hunzas living in the foothills of the Himalayas in northern Pakistan, the Georgians, Azerbaijanis and Abkhazians near Russia, the Vilacacambans in Ecuador and many others. All had exceptional longevity, with a good number of centenarians, relative freedom from disease... and a lifestyle very different from that of weWesterners. These races consumed a lot of fresh fruits and vegetables, tended towards lacto-ovo-vegetarianism and had a calorie intake just above subsistence level: they did not overeat. They had plenty of physical activity, breathed pure mountain air and lived in close-knit communities where social isolation and loneliness were virtually unknown".

The Amazing Hunza People

French continues:

"Hunzaland is a tiny country located high in the foothills of the Himalayas. It was totally isolated from the Western world until the 1920s when the British army-bearing roses, not guns – managed to make its way over the high mountain passes. In their natural, primitive state, the Hunza people exhibited perfect mental and physical health – vibrant health, in fact with many of the population living to over 100 years of age, even to 150 or more. Men at 90 years of age were known to

4

have fathered children, while women at the age of 80 looked like Western women of 40. Sickness was rare. Virtually unknown were ulcers, appendicitis, colitis, high blood pressure, heart disease or childhood illnesses. It appears that there was not a single case of cancer in the entire population"

"The people were friendly, hospitable and religious, and free of fear, hatred and jealousy. Divorce was rare and there was no juvenile delinquency. Consequently there were no jails, police or army"

"Medical studies have identified the Hunzas' natural way of eating as the major factor in their physical and mental health and wellbeing. They lived on fresh vegetables, fresh fruits, dried fruits, legumes, whole grains and goats' cheese and butter. Meat was eaten only on ceremonial occasions so it was a rarity in the diet. They did indulge in a strong grape wine. Everything was organically grown on mineral rich soils"

"In their way of life there was no refined sugar, no pasteurisation of milk, no hydrogenation of oil, no chemical fertilisers, no chlorination or fluoridation of water and no vaccination".

"They were a people of great intelligence, grace and charm, and were one of the healthiest races the world has ever seen. They still live in the same part of the world but are no longer isolated from Western influence."

Chapter 2

The History Of My Early Ancestry

My ancestors were pioneers of the first fruit shops started in Australia; actually it was in a suburb called Glebe, New South Wales. Among the first Italian immigrants from Messina to arrive on Australian shores were my grandfather's uncle, Pasquale Arena and Giovanni Tauro, a friend of his; the year they arrived was 1884 and they originally went to Hills End in Bathurst to the Gold Rush searching for gold as many European settlers did in those days. Pasquale and Giovanni didn't make a massive fortune with their gold venture but according to some relatives, did strike some gold at Bathurst, but decided to try other ways of earning a living. There weren't the opportunities available to them in those days so they had to try to find work the best way they could.

The reason the Arena family migrated to Australia was that a huge earthquake struck the City of Messina, wiping out the whole city, killing over 80,000 people, so they decided they would come to Australia for a better life with hopefully more and better opportunities. Our family and many others in those lean times left Italy with nothing and very few possessions, not knowing what was ahead of them to start a new life in a new country and speaking very little English. There were two choices at the time whether to go to America or Australia.

Some time had passed and it was now 1912 and my grandfather's parents decided to settle the whole family of seven boys and one girl in Sydney to our wonderful country, Australia. The following is a story that my mother told me many years ago -

Grandfather Percy Was A Hero

The earthquake of 1908 in Messina was so powerful that my grandfather, Percy and some members of his family nearly got killed. It all happened very quickly but Percy and his brother, Bert happened to be standing near where the ground opened up. Percy was about 12 yrs. old and Bert was about 7yrs. old at the time, when Bert nearly got swallowed up by the force and ferocity of the earthquake when the ground opened up. Luckily Percy happened to be standing nearby when he thought quickly and instinctively and immediately grabbed Bert by the hair thus saving his life. What a hero! As if that wasn't enough Percy and his older brothers realised their father Sebastiano was missing so they rushed back inside their house to find their father still trapped inside, so Percy with the help of his brothers rescued him, also saving his life.

It wasn't long after the Gold Rush venture that my grandfather's uncle Pasquale decided to open up the very first fruit shop in Sydney, which was in Glebe, New South Wales. The exact date is not sure but it was to be several years later that Pasquale's nephews, (my grandfather Percy with his brothers and father) followed and opened up fruit shops at other locations.

Fate Played A Part
In Their Survival

I think that it was fate that ALL ten members of my great- grandfather and patriarch Sebastiano and his wife and matriarch Domenica, and all their eight children survived the ravages of the 1908 earthquake in Messina which claimed the lives of 80,000 people. It was a miraculous survival, and it was their destiny that they would all come to live out their lives in their new country, Australia.

The Beginning Of Their New Life
In Australia

After the earthquake which made the Arena family and thousands of other people homeless, it is documented that the Arena family of seven sons and the only daughter, Mary, lived in barracks near Messina that were set up to accommodate people that were left homeless after the earthquake. It is said that the Italian Government and governments of neighbouring countries stepped in to help the homeless survivors of the earthquake by supplying aid, food and clothing and necessary supplies to try to make their lives a bit more comfortable.

When the Arena family first arrived in Sydney the older children were teenagers and older, led by Steve, Vince, Percy, and others, who came a few years earlier than the rest of the family to gain employment. The younger children came several years later in 1912 accompanied by their parents, Sebastiano and Domenica.

The older brothers found work wherever they could as there was this large family to support, at first setting up a furniture removals business for a short time, but they decided they may be more successful in the fruit and vegetable industry. They eventually opened up several fruit shops alongside each other in Glebe which proved to be very successful. In later years most of the brothers continued working in the fruit and vegetable industry, while two of the brothers, Roy and Bert, owned and operated taxis, all working hard determined to make it in their new country. I would like to add that all seven sons and one daughter went on to become very successful business people in their chosen occupations.

In the ensuing years that followed all the sons and daughter, Mary, eventually married and had children, grandchildren and great-grandchildren all living happily in Australia.

Chapter 3

In The 50s And 60s – That's How It Was

Let's go back to a journey in time to the 1950s. I can remember being a teenager living at home with my parents who were first generation Australian of Italian parents.

I was an only child and my mother Minnie was always cooking some very delicious Italian dishes. In those days mothers didn't work, they stayed home and looked after their families until they were old enough to stay by themselves. My mother, helped my father, Anthony Arena, in the family green grocery business, along with my Aunt Jessie and her husband, Ben Sidoti. I would also help out at weekends and sometimes after school and was about fifteen at that time.

At home It was my job to shell the peas and string the beans every weekend when Mum would do most of her cooking as she worked with Dad in our business a few days a week to help out.

For those people old enough to remember, in those days people shopped at their corner shops for groceries which sold mainly basic staples like butter, sugar, flour, canned baked beans, spaghetti, etc. There were only a few varieties of biscuits available, compared to today, which were sold from a large tin by the pound. There was also ice cream, lollies and chocolates cordials and soft drinks, and a limited amount of washing powders and cleaners as compared to today. Also their fruit and vegetables were bought at their local green grocers, like my parents' shop The owners of these stores gave personal service to their customers and served them in a very caring way, and also knew all their customers by their names.

And then something new came into our rather basic way of shopping, "THE SUPERMARKET" which revolutionised the way we shopped. The very first Supermarkets I can remember came to Australia about the early 1960's. and for those who can remember were called "Cash & Carry" stores. At first there were only two major companies and all of a sudden these supermarkets started popping up everywhere. These stores sold not only the basic staples of grocery items but hundreds of lines and then more recently hundreds of thousands of lines. Supermarkets stocked every imaginable kind of food, new snack foods, different and new kinds of tin foods; even a whole aisle devoted to pet foods. Although canned vegetables were first introduced into Australia in 1926, according to Parliamentary Research Service, it wasn't until the 1940s that canned vegetables started to appear. Canned beetroot suddenly started appearing in the traditional hamburger. By the end of the 60s canned foods were all the rage and started to take hold as many shopping trolleys could be seen overloaded with all the latest canned foods and snack foods. All of a sudden foods that were once "special treats" only eaten occasionally, were readily available every day and we kids loved the novelty of going to shop at the new Supermarkets making our mums buy all the latest chocolates and ready-packaged ice creams and ice blocks and snack foods, and many more brands and varieties of biscuits than what we were used to. We were in "Supermarket Heaven" I think it was a novelty at first going to the supermarket and asking our mums to buy all the latest snack foods and then piling them into the supermarket trolleys. These supermarkets even sold most frozen vegetables; you didn't have to go to the fruit shops to buy peas or beans or beetroot anymore because they came in a can; nor did you have to squeeze oranges any more, they came pre-packaged, ready to drink. Supermarkets became a boon to housewives as their lives became easier.

I remember being very excited about the new packaged instant mashed potato sold at the supermarket, I couldn't wait to try it. It tasted fine but proved to be expensive compared to the fresh variety. But luckily Dad still had their fruit shop and we kept eating fresh potatoes, fresh beans and all the other vegetables; but even our family switched to frozen peas; it was all too easy, to buy frozen peas instead of wasting time shelling them.

Just before the advent of "the Supermarket" it was the mid 1950s when a new exciting invention in technology started to appear in people's homes – the television set, soon known as TV. People could even buy frozen TV dinners from the Supermarket that you could be eaten in front of their TV sets; the slogan was "just heat n'eat it" how wonderful! Everybody loved it, most of all the children. TVs appeared to change the way we lived our lives as they seemed to be the focal point of peoples' living rooms. Because of TV many people preferred to spend less time cooking family meals but preferred instead to eat easy low preparation instant foods whilst watching their favourite TV programmes. Coincidentally the above device – TV and the arrival of the Supermarkets appeared at about the same time, which seemed to go hand in hand, and they were significant times that would change our diets and lifestyles forever.

Another fact comes to mind that in the mid-sixties fruit shops took a big hit then because of the above two new lifestyle changes to peoples' lives. Because TV was a very new addition to the family home, people seemed to stay home more to watch all the new and exciting TV programmes offered. Even school children couldn't wait to get home from school to watch their favourite TV shows. Because of the advent of TVs and Supermarkets housewives changed the way they shopped by being able to purchase most of their shopping needs under the one roof at their Supermarkets, such as meat, fruit and vegetables, delicatessen items, etc.

I remember my father lamenting at the time that sales of vegetables plummeted; people didn't buy fresh beetroot anymore; it was a novelty and so easy to buy it in a can. . And a lot of people didn't buy fresh potatoes for a while, they tried the instant variety because they didn't have to scrub those dirty potatoes, but they too proved too expensive for most people and so they reverted back to the fresh variety. It was at that time that frozen vegetables also appeared on supermarket shelves; consequently many people tried these and liked them, but mostly what they liked was that cooking time could be reduced and the time saved could be used for leisure activities. It was all too easy for the modern housewife. This change in diet and lifestyle was an exciting time for all the family.

Peas and beans sales dropped and business was never going to be the same after that. Fruit shops went out of vogue for a time until later on when fruit shops reinvented themselves and changed the way they sold fruit & vegies, competing with the supermarkets by selling as many items as possible including everything from delicatessen items to imported grocery items, nuts and dried fruits, etc.

To add to this, it was about the late 1960s and early 70s that the massive multinational food chains and restaurants started to invade our lives, such as Pizza Hut, McDonalds, Kentucky Fried Chicken (KFC), with many more to follow in the ensuing years. These diners started to infiltrate our suburbs and cities, making family nights out to these restaurants very appealing for parents and children alike with the tasty foods offered there.

Foods from different cultures started appearing on the restaurant scene too, such as Italian food, Lebanese, Thai etc. The winners in all this were mothers who didn't have to cook on those family nights out. People enjoyed discovering these different and interesting foods from other countries, as they were a change from their rather plain English style diet.. Take-away foods were very accessible, foods like pizza, chinese, etc. were only a phone call away where it was possible to have many kinds of fast foods delivered to your door, as it still is today.

I think it was about this time that women became liberated from the kitchen, but little did we know then that this new way of shopping, cooking, diet and lifestyle would have dire consequences to our health in the future.

And so a new era was born.

Chapter 4

Our First Experience Of Cancer In The Family

I vividly remember my first experience of Cancer in our family. I spent a lot of time at the home of my Nonna Maria, affectionately known as Nonnie, and Percy, Nonno where I learned the love of Italian food. Nonnie and Nonno were both good cooks and taught me how to cook many dishes. Most Sicilians grew up on farms in Italy so had a lot of expert knowledge about gardening and were well known for the beautiful vegetables they grew. Apart from their cooking Percy and Maria were two people who were born ahead of their time, well known for their astute business skills and just wisdom in general. I remember many people visiting Percy including family members, to obtain business advice. He was also a self-taught builder who knew many aspects of the building trade and went on to become a very successful business man.

To add to all these talents my earliest childhood memories were accompanying my parents to many weddings and functions, as we did in those days where Nonno was hired to work as an emcee. My grandfather was someone whom I idolised and looked up to and had a big influence on me. I was their first grandchild, and it was to be eight more years before they had their second grandchild, Michael, my cousin, born to my Aunt Jessie and Uncle Ben. There were to be no more grandchildren, so we were precious.

NONNO'S CANCER CAME OUT OF LEFT FIELD

I remember I was a teenager about fifteen and my grandfather was taken to hospital, after being diagnosed with bowel Cancer. I remembered that he had had a long history of constipation, and often had to resort to having enemas. He suffered much and ended up having to have 10 operations, and also having to have a colostomy which caused him a lot of grief and embarrassment and the techniques in those days were not as advanced as today. Luckily he had a loving family of my grandmother (Nonnie) and my mother and Aunt Jessie who worked around the clock attending to his colostomy bag, which regularly needed attention. This routine went on for several years which took its toll on all of them, but they were very emotionally strong women and did whatever they had to do by caring for him and trying to make his life bearable.

There was no chemotherapy in those days but radiation which they called Cobalt which was very harsh on the body. He ended up going in and out of hospital having daily Cobalt treatments and endured 5 years of suffering, but unfortunately succumbed to the disease and finally died an agonizing death. His death had a profound impact on me, as I saw him suffering and dying in a horrific, painful and degrading way. He was only 64, leaving my grandmother alone who was also 64.

Nonnie went on to live another 34 years until she was 98 years; she had a big influence on me and was blessed with very healthy longevity and it was wonderful to have her in our lives for such a long time.

Percy's Siblings Died Young

My grandfather's five brothers also died rather young. Two others died from bowel cancer, Roy who was 64 and Joe who was 70; the eldest brother Steve, died from TB. All five brothers didn't make it to 70yrs; there was also one sister, Mary, who died very young at 62 from a heart attack; her twin, Bert, died very young, also from a heart attack at age 56. Only one brother, Leo, lived to the ripe old age of 93; he was lucky. In his later years he apparently had heart trouble, but actually died from cancer also. There wasn't much information about cholesterol in those days, and having a healthy diet and lifestyle were unknown.

After seeing my grandfather's horrible end I was determined that I didn't want to see any more family members die in this way so I started to research diets and longevity and why some people die young and others live to old age, virtually disease-free.

It wasn't until many years later; I wondered if they had known about diet and cholesterol and blood pressure, etc. would they have lived much longer instead of having their lives cut so short? It was about this time that I started to take an interest in healthy eating and researched the many diseases so prevalent in today's society and I began reading about health and diets and longevity being tied into good eating and a healthy lifestyle and regular exercise and foods that were healthy and foods that were not. I realised that the typical Italian diet was partly responsible for my ancestors' bad health, and my own bad health, due to a lack of fibre and high in salt.

Their diets consisted of too many dishes containing a lot of cheese, (partly responsible for cholesterol) which is used in many Italian dishes, too much meat in the diet, cured meats like salami and mortadella, and prosciutto, etc. (which contain nitrates, nitrites and much salt) were eaten on a regular basis and probably too much bread and pasta, and salty foods like olives and anchovies, capers, etc. etc. Salt featured heavily in Italian cooking in those days and sadly still does today. I cannot single out Italian Cuisine as being the culprit, because most other cultures do NOT use salt sparingly either. Salads were basic and vegetables would have been overcooked; (the way many people cooked their vegetables in those times and still do) The typical southern Italian diet is still prevalent today in people coming from that region, and whilst they are enjoying what they eat are not totally unaware of some of the unhealthy elements of their diet., and it could be killing them? Don't get me wrong – I still love Italian cooking, I was brought up on it, but I believe that the recipes can be modified to incorporate more leafy green vegetables cooked in a healthy way, with lots of creative salads to balance

19

out the rather unhealthier dishes. Italian Cuisine is very flavourful but it is not one of the healthiest.

Coffee featured heavily in the Italian diet in those times, in fact many people today are also hooked on coffee, a habit that most people find hard to give up; it is a coffee culture; coffee shops are popping up everywhere. All the above foods are hard to digest and can cause constipation, which is a correlation with bowel Cancer, a fact that was to come to light many years later.

Better Times Ahead

It was now 1966 and about this time that I met my husband and soulmate Joseph. He came at a time when I needed cheering up after the loss of my grandfather and my grandmother always said that God sent Joe to me. Joe also came from an ethnic background; his mother Millie, was Lebanese, from whose family I was to learn much about the Lebanese cuisine and his father Gaetano, better known as Tom was also Sicilian from Italy. Our wedding was an Italian style lavish affair with 400 guests (just the family and a few friends).

A few years later our children were born, first came a son, Tommy, and then, two years later, a daughter, Melissa, who are the absolute best children anyone could ever want, and adored by everyone.

Suddenly My Life Changed

Just when life was ticking along nicely and our children were growing; I think they were about 11 and 9 respectively, when I was involved in a car accident which resulted in me getting a whiplash and the shock of that accident brought on what was the beginning of very painful rheumatoid arthritis (autoimmune disease where the body attacks itself) causing swollen painful joints, hands and feet and ankles and neck pain and later a frozen shoulder. This arthritis was to plague me for many years to come and my health was never the same after that. Because of the whiplash my neck was painful and I needed regular chiropractic treatments which went on for years.

I first consulted medical practitioners who prescribed the usual non- steroidal anti-inflammatory drugs, which worked for a while, and then I seemed to be immune to them and they also upset my stomach. Finally a friend suggested I visit a naturopath, which I did, and he sat down with me for an hour and went through my diet and suggested I give up meat, wheat and dairy as they were very acidic, indicating that acid foods can cause rheumatic symptoms and if I cut those out I would feel better. At first they were hard to give up as I was used to a very high animal protein diet, but it made me be more creative in the dishes that I prepared. He also instructed me to buy a juice extractor and make a juice every morning and drink more water and buy a water filter; instructions I obeyed and still practise to this day. I was desperate to get rid of the pain and these practices seemed to work for a few years and I was feeling much better.

Several years later I had another trauma in another traffic incident which gave me a frozen shoulder, and not having much physical activity at the time, plus the fact I was also traumatised from the accident, probably contributed to this condition. This frozen shoulder stayed with me for several years and it seemed that I had a lot of inflammation in my body, but I was able to keep it all under control with a healthy diet and regular exercise like hydrotherapy and walking and shoulder exercises.

Chapter 5

Cancer Was Never Far Away

The next person to be struck down with cancer was my dear mother-in-law, Millie, with whom I had a great relationship. She was always a very happy woman who loved entertaining; her husband, Tom was also very skilled in the kitchen and loved cooking sicilian recipes, which he remembered from his childhood. He had a lot of experience cooking as he served as a cook in the army during World War 11. The two of them made a good combination and their home was always open to their family and the many friends they had accumulated over the years. Millie loved cooking for them and her table was always bursting with delicious Lebanese and Italian dishes from both of their cultures, and she was also renowned for her baked dinners and apple pies. Millie, being of Lebanese heritage, loved eating all the rich traditional foods that she was used to preparing not knowing that one day her diet would have an adverse effect on her health.

Her death was sudden and swift and totally out of left field. The year was 1984 and I can remember vividly we were holidaying in Queensland with our two children who were 15 and 13 at the time; on our return my father phoned us to say that Millie had been admitted to hospital with pneumonia and upper respiratory problems. At first we weren't really perturbed thinking that it wasn't serious, but the doctors were treating her for pneumonia and she wasn't responding to the treatment they were giving her. Clearly she was not getting any better and still feeling very unwell when the doctors finally decided to conduct an Ultra Sound on her, and to our horror it revealed that she had the Big C. We were shocked to the core; this news was devastating for all of us, especially for Joe and his brother, Anthony, who were very devoted to their mother.

Millie was diagnosed with cancer, but the doctors didn't know where the primary cancer had started and it had now reached the lungs and spreading. Her cancer was very advanced and now terminal. She only lasted three more months, dying on the 12th April which was her brother Mick's birthday and also around Easter time, making her death even more significant, ensuring that on every anniversary of her death she would never be forgotten. It was a date firmly fixed in our minds and one we have always remembered. She was only 72.

Tom's Cancer Also Came Out Of Left Field

As Millie's death came to us all as an unexpected shock, my father-in-law, Tom, now a widower, found it hard to cope for a while and the loneliness that accompanies losing a loved one, especially one's life partner, learned to adapt to his new situation and drew on his cooking experience whilst serving in the army in the World War 2 and along with the household duties was able to look after himself quite competently. He kept himself busy playing golf and enjoyed regular outings going to the races and socialising with friends.

He also continued with his hobby of growing orchids; at one stage he had 500 orchids growing in the special orchid enclosure that he himself erected. At this point Joe and I decided we would like to move house closer to his dad so he could spend more time with him. Joe and I were pleased we made the timely move as he was able to visit his dad more often. Tom liked to talk about old times and politics and life in general and it was good to see them both bonding again. Tom was 72 when Millie died but went on to live another seventeen years before he himself finally succumbed to Cancer.*

Cancer Strikes Again

Tom, unlike Millie, followed a mostly vegetarian diet with lots of fruit and vegetables and legumes and only ate a small amount of meat occasionally, and did not drink alcohol or smoke, even though he had smoked heavily in his youth and continued to do so for the next 50 years, finally giving it up after much pressure from family and his doctor warning that he wouldn't live much longer if he continued to smoke, his lungs already weakened by the many years of smoking.

Even with his history of heavy smoking, his tireless energy and longevity was a testimony to his healthy diet and lifestyle.

Tom's death was also sad and unexpected. I remember it well – the year was 2001. One evening he collapsed and fell to the floor and was coughing up blood. Fortunately he was wearing a health monitor around his neck which immediately connected to the Head Office when he pressed the button which probably saved his life as he was unable to pull himself up from the floor. Very soon we were contacted and an ambulance arrived quickly; the paramedics were able to enter Tom's home through a back door which just by chance was luckily left unlocked. He was then taken to the nearest hospital and extensive tests were carried out on him; he had had issues with his prostate and the doctors discovered he had prostate cancer.

They operated on him and removed the prostate but found that after further tests the cancer had spread to his bones. He had no hope of surviving as the cancer was well advanced and terminal as well. He spent the next ten weeks in several hospitals and finally succumbed to the disease on 9th December, 2001. Coincidentally, Millie and Tom died from cancer in a similar way; both lasted only three months, Millie died on her brother, Mick's birthday and Tom died on my Aunt Jessie's birthday; dates that make sure we don't forget them.

My Father's Blood Disease

The next person to be struck down with a deadly disease was my father, Tony. It was Aplastic Anaemia; although it is not cancer, is closely related to it, and may be associated with certain cancers especially those affecting the bone marrow, and that it is capable of killing the person afflicted with it. The disease causes the bone marrow not to produce red cells, white cells and platelets in the blood nor sufficient new cells to replenish blood cells. The symptoms are debilitating in that he was always very tired and pale looking and often breathless. He was kept alive by the medications and blood transfusions he was taking for about ten years.

During that time he would get very low on energy and my mother Minnie, had to take him to hospital at regular intervals for blood transfusions. These transfusions usually took about 2-3 days. He would have to go to hospital every 2 months and then these transfusions became more and more often until the organs in his body started to shut down and the doctors could do no more for him, when he finally succumbed to the disease. He was only 72; making my mother a widow at the young age of 69. Mum lived another thirteen years, dying from kidney disease at the age of 81.

Chapter 6

Hope At Hopewood

It was about this time that my frozen shoulder was causing me a lot of pain, that I had heard about a health retreat called Hopewood situated in Wallacia, NSW. It is a country style, semi-rural health retreat situated in the peaceful foothills of the Blue Mountains where people go to unwind while at the same time learn about Natural Health guidelines which means healing diseases naturally and not with medication. Whilst there I met many like-minded people, some were battling obesity, others were there to detoxify their systems and all the guests were there to get educated on a healthy diet and the causes of many of our faulty diet and lifestyle diseases;

Hopewood guests also attended cooking lessons on how to prepare healthy vegetarian dishes. Whilst there I also went for walks, attended yoga and stretch classes and swam in the heated pool doing aqua aerobic exercises, or had one of the many types of massages available. Whilst I was there I also had various consultations with experienced naturopaths who told me about the deadly nightshade vegetables from the Solanacea family like tomatoes, eggplants, capsicums and white potatoes and also vinegar, which caused a lot of acidity and were responsible for a lot of arthritic pain. I also learned that to obtain good health and to eliminate inflammation from the body we should aim to eat an alkaline diet, which is a well-balanced ratio of 80% alkaline foods to 20% acid foods. Acid foods are meat, dairy and grains and alkaline foods are fruits and vegetables.

I had two stays within two years at Hopewood Health Retreat and during my stays there learned that diseases of arthritis and most other diseases can be cured or relieved without any harmful pharmaceutical medications and their nasty side-effects, just by adhering to a semi-vegetarian or vegetarian diet, and only drinking healthy drinks and filtered water. using "food as medicine" under Natural Health Guidelines.

There were many talks given at Hopewood given by very knowledgeable naturopaths who knew their stuff. They said that most of our diseases are caused by a faulty diet and lifestyle and too many take away foods and a reliance on convenience foods causing a toxic overload on the intestines, a self-poisoning of the digestive system. I later learned that students studying Naturopathy have to undertake extensive study on Diet and Nutritional studies to become naturopaths, about 300 to 400 hours, compared to medical orthodox doctors who study only about six hours of diet and nutrition.

Many of the guests at Hopewood were put on juice fasts or delicious vegetarian style eating to detoxify their systems. Meat and dairy foods were not allowed at Hopewood or any junk or processed foods were off limits. Tea and coffee and alcohol were not allowed also. The diet consisted of legumes, nuts, fruit and vegetables all cooked in a delicious way by the Hopewood chefs.

Whilst at Hopewood, there were several talks on health and during that time I met health professionals and Life Coaches who advocated Food Combining for optimum health.

Food Combining, a practice I had not heard about where you eat animal proteins with other vegetables instead of with starches or rice or pasta for better digestion and consequently better elimination and bowel action. At first I found this practice very hard to do as we have all been brought up to eat potatoes or rice with meat or chicken, also the health practitioners advised not to drink with meals and wait at least one to two hours before or after meals before eating any fruit.

After both my stays at Hopewood I returned home feeling much better after all that healthy food and country air. But I still had the frozen shoulder and was to have it for a few more years. After putting up with the pain for a while, I finally had an MRI done of my shoulder and found that I had a torn rotator-cuff, which cannot be fixed solely with diet. Most people have surgery on it but I refused as I have had other operations for arthritis, and wanted to see if I could heal my shoulder problem naturally, without surgery. Some people have fixed their shoulder problems using natural therapies, such as massage and appropriate exercises, whilst there are others who are in a lot of pain and have to resort to shoulder surgery. At the moment I am trying the alternative things like massage, diet, and a hand pulley attached to a door or wooden beam, which I use several times a day, and hydrotherapy swimming which is in a water temperature of 34 degrees, making exercise much easier and less painful. These methods are proving successful for me and I have noticed a marked improvement with more strength in both my shoulders as I stay focused, and also try not to lift any unnecessary heavy bags whilst shopping.

NOTE. Since the time of writing I am sorry to say that Hopewood has recently closed its doors to the public, due to occupancy being low in numbers. Hopewood Health Retreat first opened its doors in 1960 and from then on over the many years of successful operation catered to and healed many people with health ailments or just people who wanted to get away from it all in a healthy manner and relaxed atmosphere.

However, Hopewood still wants to continue its message on Natural Health guidelines. To help people adopt and maintain Hopewood's health message, there are five content themes on their site. Firstly there is the LIFESTYLE section, and then the HEAL section, and then there are the MOVE, NURTURE and EAT sections.

Go to hopewood.com.au to get immediate access to Hopewood's Natural Health philosophy.

Chapter 7

My Cancer Story
I Didn't See It Coming

Two years before my actual cancer diagnosis I had some unusual and rather worrying symptoms that I was rather concerned about. I had been experiencing constant fatigue, continued unexplained weight loss, which went on for about 12 months, despite eating a substantial diet, and very low anaemia levels, accompanied by persistent constant chronic fatigue, a symptom I had been plagued with on and off for many years, also a painful swollen lymph node in the groin. This swelling resembled a hernia but turned out not to be anything serious at the time. There was also a constant, noticeable diarrhoea-like change in bowel motions, something I had never experienced. I thought at this stage maybe I should see a specialist. I did so and he ordered me to go to hospital to conduct tests. For four days some gruelling tests were conducted on me, but at that stage the tests revealed nothing, however my doctor had suspected lymphoma all along but as reflected by all the tests performed on me, there were no visible signs of any lymphoma at that time. In retrospect I realise now that cancer was brewing and growing insidiously inside my body and I, oblivious of the fact went home from hospital very relieved that all tests were negative, but did not in any way suspect what was to come twelve months later when I was to receive the shock of my life.

I didn't see it coming

It all started back in August, 2010; I was 65 at the time and had been cleaning out my fridge and wiping the shelves down, when that night I noticed my hand and arm were a bit sore. The next day my right arm started to swell, especially around the elbow area. At first I thought I had strained my arm with overuse and too much cleaning. Before I knew it, and over a period of some weeks my right hand was swollen and my lower arm and elbow had blown up like a balloon into twice its original size into a very large arm so much so that I could hardly get any jumpers over it. The sight of my arm was very scary.

At first I consulted my local GP and later a Hand Specialist surgeon, both of whom could not find anything wrong with me, so I came home and wondered what on earth could this swelling mean, not knowing what was ahead of me. Then during the last week in September I developed excruciating nerve pain in the middle of my right hand causing me a week of sleepless nights.

It wasn't until the long weekend in October 2010 that my son came to dinner and I told him that he had better take me to the nearest hospital as I couldn't stand the pain in my hand any longer, and it was gradually getting worse and I thought, well this is something serious but I have no clue as to what it might be?

I stayed in hospital for 16 days as the doctors put me through every test imaginable. Finally they did a lymph node biopsy under my arm and discovered that I had Non-Hodgkins Lymphoma, which is cancer of the lymph nodes and the swollen elbow was caused by a malignant tumour growing in there. How confronting it was when we were told this news. Following the biopsy the doctors wanted to investigate further to see if the cancer had spread, and ordered a PET scan, which scans the whole body looking for abnormalities, and tests revealed that I had Stage 2 Bone Cancer in the left shoulder as well. My heart sank as I wasn't expecting to be diagnosed with not only one type of cancer but life threatening Stage 2 Bone Cancer as well, and the worst possible consequences from cancer treatment that were to follow.

My husband and son were with me when we were told the scary news and it filled us all with terror, especially as my doctor told me that because I had the bone cancer in my shoulder I would have to have very strong drugs with chemotherapy and I would gradually lose my hair and I had better buy a wig immediately as I would start to lose my hair after the third treatment, until it all would fall out completely, half way through the treatment. This news rocked me to the core – what? No hair? Would it grow back again? How was I going to cope? This news was very confronting, and I had vowed that if I ever got cancer,

I would never have chemotherapy, as it was against my beliefs, but it seemed I had no choice and had to go along with the doctor's advice that the cancer was life-threatening and that I wouldn't survive without it.

Confronted With My Own Mortality

All of a sudden like never before, I was confronted with my own mortality, confused and scared, not knowing what was ahead of me. Would I survive or would I die? How long would I last? My doctor recommended that I must have three months of intensive chemotherapy treatment with strong drugs administered via chemotherapy, which entailed a minimum dose to start, with each session of chemo. lasting 5-6 hours. These sessions were the minimum dose of chemotherapy usually prescribed which consisted of six treatments These sessions were to be on the basis of two weeks apart, the duration of which lasted twelve weeks in all.. My doctor told me if the chemotherapy treatment didn't work I was to then have some radiation.

With that horrific possibility I thought "I certainly hope not"

Well, I thought, I am going to try and rid myself of all this cancer, have the minimum course of orthodox drugs as prescribed by my cancer specialist of the six sessions of chemotherapy, and get out of the chemotherapy ward as quickly as possible, and armed with the knowledge I had gained over the years going to Hopewood Health Retreat and doing extensive reading on many books and health articles on diet, and its relationship with disease and longevity.

However, friends and relations were puzzled and questioned how could I possibly be struck down with Cancer when I was already on a very healthy diet and had been for many years. But I had a hunch that even though I ate the right foods, my digestive system must still be severely compromised and clogged with toxins (a back-log of waste) and I was right!

If ever there was a time to put my knowledge about food and diet to the test, then this was it! This knowledge had enabled me to recreate my own diet with healthy but tasty recipes, and I adopted a semi-vegetarian, mostly plant-based diet, and lots of salads, along with drinking lots of filtered water only, and put my knowledge of proper food combining to the test.

I then realised there is a strong correlation between a toxic digestive system that contains impacted faecal matter that sits on the walls of the intestines rotting and toxifying, could this toxic state possibly cause cancer cells to grow. Having spoken to people with different types of cancer confide that they have long standing bowel and constipation issues, along with headaches mostly caused by bad circulation and stodgy blood that is lacking oxygen, through lack of fibre and the correct fluids.

My First Day Of Chemotherapy

My first treatment of chemotherapy was very scary and confronting. I arrived early and saw people streaming into the chemo ward with varying stages of chemotherapy, some had already lost their hair, some wore scarves and others wore wigs, who were mostly women. Talking to patients in the chemo ward were also people who had reoccurrences of cancer and had to endure more chemo treatment, with some women I met had to endure the degrading single and double mastectomy surgery.

Initially my first chemo treatment was scary at first, not knowing what was about to happen. First, I was given some pain killers to deaden the pain of the cannula as it was being inserted into my arm; the cannula was attached to a large bag of the awful cocktail of poisonous drugs (chemo) that was pumped into my system. I was so traumatised that I couldn't even turn my head to look at this bag of poison entering my body. I think that on that first day of treatment I said several Rosaries along with my strong faith in God and devotion to Our Lady I suddenly had an epiphany moment and vowed that if I was able to beat this cancer I certainly wanted to tell other people and write a book about it.

My first treatment lasted 6 hours, starting at 9.30a.m. and finishing at 3.30 in the afternoon, and I was to have 5 more equally long treatments two weeks apart. At that point I resolved again to get my chemo. treatments over with and get out of that chemotherapy ward as soon as possible. I did not want to be there!

Whilst I was enduring my first chemotherapy treatment I had a lot of hope and a good feeling that I might be able to cure these two life-threatening cancers quickly. I started to tell myself over and over again that I must still have a backlog of faecal matter in my intestines, rotting and toxifying, which could possibly be the culprit which caused my two cancers to grow and multiply??

Combined with all the knowledge I had acquired through extensive reading about living healthily and having two visits at Hopewood Health Retreat, where I learned so much about diet being related to disease and Food Combining principles, I would put all my knowledge into a dietary regime which excluded any foods with sugar, eating only all the "good stuff" and only drinking natural fluids and pure water, I immediately started on my already rather strict regime by detoxifying and ridding my digestive tract of accumulated waste.

After the first chemo. treatment and up to the sixth and final treatment, I never experienced the dreadful fatigue other people spoke of, and always had a lot of energy when I returned home from treatment that I would go for a walk and was able to cook dinner for my husband without a problem. I did feel slightly nauseous though throughout the treatment, realising that the chemo destroys the taste buds and certain foods that I normally like were distasteful and made me feel ill.

Luckily for me, I was NEVER actually physically sick, and was able to cook dinner every night whilst having chemotherapy treatment, possibly due to the healthy and detoxifying diet that I had undertaken..I believe there are many people who after enduring many chemotherapy sessions, are unable to eat or even cook for some time because they are so physically ill. Chemotherapy may kill bad cells but also destroys good cells.

Hair Loss Was Devastating

My Doctor had warned me that I would likely lose my hair and I should purchase a wig immediately, as hair loss can start gradually and then fall out rapidly. I took his advice and bought my wig and the prediction by the doctor proved to be correct and by the third treatment my very thick hair started to thin out at first and then by the fourth and sixth treatment it all came out in clumps, leaving me completely bald! I was devastated by the total loss of my hair over this period of time as I was forced to wear my wig for vanity's sake and the ensuing six months proved to be the longest and most testing time of my life. At the same time for good measure, as if I already had enough horrible side-effects to contend with, I had to endure painful mouth ulcers, the likes of which I have never experienced in my life. Fortunately for me they only lasted for a few weeks.

Immediate Improvement
After 1ˢᵗ Chemo Treatment

The week after each chemo treatment I had to consult with my doctor , and even immediately the week after the first treatment, my doctor, on examining me to my and his delight, exclaimed that he COULDN'T find any swellings in any of my lymph nodes, considering when I first presented with symptoms of lymphoma a month previously, I had multiple enlarged lymph node swellings in my right axilla (armpit) and mediastinum and right hilum, ranging in size of 2cm to 3cm x 5.5.2cm as well as many other abnormal enlarged lymph nodes in the entire chest wall and throughout the entire lymphatic system. My first report also showed Thyroid nodules were present in the left lobe of the thyroid gland.

But then almost miraculously, on the same day as my first consultation after my first chemo. session my doctor could not find any evidence of the tumour in my elbow. He was shocked but delighted with these fantastic results and said he was very happy with me but I still had to continue and finish the next five treatments that he had originally prescribed. I told him that I was on a very healthy diet and he told me to "keep going with your diet" The same reaction followed on the second, third, fourth, fifth and sixth treatments. My doctor still could not find any lymph node swellings or any tumour, nor was there was any evidence of ANY cancer anywhere in my body.

Sudden Shocking Side-Effects

After I had completed the six prescribed chemo sessions, I awoke one morning and found I was not going to escape more horrific nasty side effects from the treatment, I awoke to find I couldn't get out of bed, because of chronic fatigue, and had intermittent diarrhoea and had trouble keeping weight on. I realised these were the scary side-effects from the chemotherapy treatment. To add to all this, my weight plummeted from my already small frame of 49 kilos down to 43 kilos and I hated the fact that my clothes were falling off me. I was like a zombie and these horrendous, scary side effects went on for a month.

In the mornings I would drag myself out of bed and eat a little breakfast and then go back to bed as I had no energy to do anything else; I just wanted to sleep all the time. Most afternoons I would struggle out of bed again and cook dinner for myself and my husband. I was, however able to eat dinner every night without much nauseousness and trying to keep up my strength and gain a little weight. These symptoms dragged on for a month and I felt scared. How long was this going to go on? What was going to happen to me? Was I going to survive? Finally I consulted a naturopath who prescribed a powder to bulk the bowel and another powder to normalise and solidify bowel motions. This treatment worked almost at once and to my relief I started to feel much better and gradually began to gain weight, still adhering to the diet.

A Miraculous Recovery

Finally, after the sixth treatment my doctor requested that I have another PET scan to see if there were still signs of cancer or if it had spread to other organs. To my utter surprise and delight he read the report results to me via email and it read like this "the malignant lymphoma in your elbow has resolved and the Scan shows no sign of any more cancer. The cancer in your bone is all clear. You had made a remarkable recovery. Excellent!"

I am happy to report that my hair did grow back thick and strong as it was before the treatment, but it took about seven months to do so.

I would like to think that my cancer recovery was in record time and I attribute it all to the fact that I only needed a minimum of six sessions of chemo. but most importantly my perseverance and confidence in my healthy diet.

Chapter 8

Food Combining – An Important Tool In Combating Cancer

Food Combining is a rather unknown and little publicised, but effective method of eating used for good digestion and better elimination of bowel movements, and gaining popularity with many diet-oriented, naturopathic practitioner consultants. Without proper food combining I think I would not have got the successful results I obtained with my cancer diet. In our western diet we are used to eating protein with potatoes or rice, drinking with meals, and eating fruit straightaway after meals. Food Combining contradicts all this. Food combining is based on the concept that different enzymes are needed to digest protein and different enzymes are needed to digest starches. If the two are mixed together they can clash and food ferments in the gut causing embarrassing flatulence, bad digestion and can also disrupt sleep patterns as I can attest to. Bad food combining also causes poorly digested food which can cause constipation and too few badly formed stools.

I, like most of us were brought up to eat many different combinations of food, sometimes two starches, two proteins in one meal, drinking what we like, then fruit or desserts eaten straight away. Help! What an assault on our poor digestive systems!

Food Combining has made me creative, for example when looking for a vegetable to substitute potatoes, pumpkin etc., I discovered a vegetable called swede, a vegetable that doesn't have the full starch like potatoes, etc.; when boiled and mashed it is a good substitute. A swede is also called a Rutabaga. In Australia, they are available all year round. There is another good vegetable which is a substitute for potatoes and that is celeriac. Celeriac is usually a knobbly, gnarly-looking root vegetable, and is a seasonal delight found in the winter months from May to December (in Australia). Celeriac also has less starch than white potatoes so is suitable to team up with proteins. They can be baked like you would cook potatoes in the oven. Carrots are also a good substitute for potatoes, as they are lower in carbohydrates and are less starchy and combine well with most vegetables.

Alternatively, protein foods, that is animal proteins or legume proteins, can be teamed up with a pile of leafy green vegetables, which are perfect for digestion and health and weight loss.

Starches should be eaten separately, for example a rice meal or a pasta meal should be eaten with the right combinations of vegetables like leafy greens and maybe carrots. When eating a starch meal, no animal protein or legumes should be eaten with starches. Two proteins should also not be eaten together at the same meal like meat or chicken with legumes, as this disrupts digestion and good sleeping patterns. When eating a legume meal, it should not be eaten with rice or heavy starches as they clash, also disrupting sleep and digestion patterns. From my own experience, I find that when I eat a properly combined vegetarian meal I get a good night's sleep and it is accompanied with good digestion.

Eating a heavy meal just before going to bed or a improperly combined meal can sometimes cause bad dreams and nightmares. Good food combining often prevents this from happening. A properly combined meal should facilitate a good night's sleep – provided there are no worrying thoughts or stresses on your mind, and you are able to switch off your brain and go to sleep.

Insomniacs can be greatly helped with combining the right foods. There are certain foods I find that help people to sleep well, and foods that give disruptive sleep. For instance if I don't eat leafy greens at night I don't sleep; if I have eaten out at a restaurant and couldn't get the right vegetables or salads, that night I may not sleep well or if I eat too much animal protein for dinner that night I may not sleep; also eating late at night or when eating out at dinner time, and eating different rich foods to which one is not accustomed can also play havoc with good sleeping patterns. Also restaurants tend to over-salt food or use additives in their sauces as in some Asian cuisines which can seriously disrupt sleep. Sometimes it is the price to pay for a GOOD night out.

Drinking With Meals
Is A No No

I don't drink with meals only at breakfast time; it is best to drink most fluids in the morning or during the day, not late afternoon or at night-time as you have to make too many trips to the bathroom during the night, when fluids are needed the most. Fluids dilute the digestive juices interfering with the digestion of solid foods. Fruit should be eaten at least one hour before or two hours after a meal, especially at dinner time. All melons should be eaten separately, on their own or with other melons such as rockmelon, honeydew and watermelon, etc. but not eaten with other fruits. Other fruits such as acid fruits should be eaten separately such as oranges, pineapple, mandarins, kiwi fruit, strawberries and passionfruit. Then there are sub-acid fruits which should be eaten separately such as most stone fruits like apricots, plums, grapes, pears, nectarines, berries, cherries and mangos. If fluids are eaten too soon after a meal they sit on top of the foods in the stomach and ferment.

Food Combining practices have given me a feeling of exhilaration and well-being, with tons of energy, something I never experienced when I ate poorly combined foods, and people are continuing to tell me how well I look. Food combining is also excellent for weight loss as it enables people to eat a lot of the correct food without starving, and a feeling of fullness, giving good digestion and better bowel function. Proper food combining has the added bonus of giving a feeling of well-being and an alertness and clarity of mind, along with a positive attitude, not a foggy brain which often contributes to not having the ability to focus on everyday duties.

Depression And Bi-Polar Disease Can Be Linked To Diet

Health experts are finally discovering that there IS a link between patients suffering from bouts of depression and bi-polar disease, whose diets are severely lacking in green and leafy vegetables, with too much dependency on take away and junk foods and soft drinks. From my point of view I agree with that reasoning that the foods we eat have an impact on our moods, whether depressed or happy, and I find that if I eat foods with trans-fats and no green or leafy vegetables, it is easy to feel depressed. Perhaps if doctors learned more about the correct foods to eat and then prescribe them to depressed and bi-polar patients, instead of solely over-medicating them with pills and tranquillisers, they may get more successful results.

How To Get A Good Night's Sleep

When trying to go to sleep at night look for foods that contain melatonin, a naturally occurring sleep hormone contained in leafy greens, legumes, omega-3 fish, etc. I believe that a good serving of watermelon two hours after dinner is a good sleep inducer, it usually ensures long relaxing sleep, as it contains mostly water which helps digestion. There is something about watermelon which relaxes the muscles, hydrates cells and balances the Ph in our bodies, as well as containing fibre and other vitamins and also hydrates the skin.

On many occasions when we dine out for lunch and have eaten a large meal, dinner time comes around and we naturally aren't very hungry, so for dinner we eat a bowl of nutritious legume or vegetable soup followed by a good serve of watermelon two hours later, and then just before retiring drink a large glass of warm water with a squeeze of lemon, waiting at least one hour after eating fruit. We find that these measures help to digest the heavy meal eaten at lunchtime and usually give restful sleep.

Listed below are my twelve tips for a good night's sleep.

1. No coffee after 4.00pm or anything containing caffeine, cola drinks, or chocolate or chocolate desserts or biscuits, etc.
2. If you are accustomed to having bad dreams or nightmares, the solution to that is to try to eat a properly combined meal e.g. fresh fish with omega-3 oils such as salmon, ocean trout or chicken with appropriately combined vegetables, (no rice or potatoes) for better digestion and restful

sleep will follow. I find that eating a good tranquilising vegetable is Chinese broccoli; it is bitter but very calming.

3. Avoid eating meals too late at night or when dining out as that can be a problem and then going straight to bed on a full stomach means food sits in the stomach and can't be digested, so disrupting sleep. An ideal time to eat dinner is between 6 and 7pm.

4. Avoid eating too many heavy rich meals and rich desserts. Eat fresh fruit instead. Try eating small amounts of animal protein like chicken or fish with leafy greens and salads. Eating a meal comprising a lot of meat can sometimes disrupt sleep and digestion. A properly combined protein-free meal also helps to get restful sleep.

5. Try to limit computer use before retiring; the lights of the computer can act as stimulants so keeping you awake; at the same time try to keep all phones and other electronic devices out of the bedroom.

6. Try not to engage in stimulating conversations or fiery discussions close to bedtime, save them for the daytime, if possible.

7. Drink a large glass of warm water with a squeeze of lemon just before bed.

8. To prepare yourself for sleep take a book or magazine to read to do a crossword or two, so making you drowsy.

9. It is important to have the right pillow for sleeping, especially those who are prone to headaches. Invest in a good chiropractic pillow which is good for

supporting the neck and head whilst sleeping. The mattress we sleep on is also very important and should be considered; how old is it? is it a bit tired and flat? It might be time to update with a good quality comfortable mattress. Mattresses need to be turned over and rotated every few months to even out the wear, which enables them to support the spine and then mattresses will last much longer. Curtains and window coverings should also be considered; heavy drapes and sheers that can be closed at night to provide a totally dark environment or blinds or shutters that provide total darkness. These measures can improve sleep patterns enormously!

10. Try to switch off the brain from any stresses or worrying thoughts as these can disrupt sleep.

11. Exercise is a good tranquiliser; try to have at least thirty minutes exercise every day out in the fresh air, if possible, be it walking, swimming, yoga or tai chi or qigong or taking part in sport, or going to the gym etc.

12. Some medications like Prednisolone etc. can sleepless nights, so be aware of any medications taken. Throw away those sleeping pills as these can have worrying side effects?

There are several books written on Food Combining and to better explain Food Combining principles in depth there is an excellent book available on the subject, called "Food Combining" by Tim Spong and Vicki Peterson.

Chapter 9

Tai Chi And Qigong – An Important Modality

Not long after my cancer diagnosis my neighbour and good friend, Pauline Huang came to visit me. Pauline hails from Beijing but has been living in Australia for many years now and is a Tai Chi and QiGong instructor with the Confucius Institute, Sydney University. She explained that I needed to do some light Qigong exercises, not Tai Chi as they were too strenuous for me. She explained that my lymphatic system was very sluggish with the large tumour that had grown in it; with lack of correct exercises and lack of activity, along with toxicity, I had stifled my lymphatic system, and now it had choked me. With that good advice I started to do Qigong exercises regularly and felt better knowing they were helping me. I also suffered from headaches and found that the movements from QiGong helped minimise the regular headaches I was getting.

In those early days of uncertain times of which way my health was heading, just after my cancer diagnosis I found that Tai Chi and Qigong helped my mental state as well as my physical state, which also played a part in my rapid recovery from cancer.

Every day, even now, I make it a practise to do some form of exercise, whether it be Qigong or stretching exercises, along with walking or hydrotherapy pool exercises. Exercise is a must to treat cancer as it is relaxing to the body and there is no substitute for getting out in the fresh air walking, especially by the sea if possible.

Many people believe meditation is beneficial in assisting cancer recovery and I can't argue with that.

The Great Grand Master Kellen Chia, from the Tai Chi Society writes:

Overview

"Tai chi and Qigong are ancient practices that have led to improved health, fitness, wellbeing and longevity for countless individuals up to the present time. They both cultivate the Qi, also spelt Chi – the life energy that flows through the body's energy pathways—by combining movement, breathing and meditation. Tai chi and QiGong have in common the same basic property (Qi) the same fundamental principle (relaxation) and the same fundamental method (slowness). Tai Chi's other principles, methods and applications are distinct to Qigong regarding how the form is practised, how the energy is manipulated and how the body posture is conditioned."

What Is Qi?

"Qi is the animating power that permeates the universe and all living things. It is a basis for traditional Chinese Medicine (ATM) – Qi flows throughout the body's energy pathways, or meridians, to help maintain essential health. The body is unwell when the flow of Qi becomes stagnant or blocked, whereas a free flowing and balanced Qi energizes the organs, systems and cells."

What Is Qigong?

"QiGong literally means "life energy work" – a way of working with the life energy. It is a healing art, a way of cultivating physical, spiritual, emotional and physical health that originated in China about seven thousand years ago, widely practised by the shaman priests during that primitive era. Qigong is part of Traditional Chinese Medicine and was first detailed in an ancient Chinese medical text book – the Huang Di Nei or Yellow emperor's Inner Canon – that has been regarded as the fundamental doctrinal source for Chinese medicine for well over two millennia and is still in use today. Subsequent Chinese medical books published in antiquity also reveal detailed theory and the clinical practice of qigong procedures for treating disease and enhancing health. The art of Qigong can be practised as physical movement that incorporates breathing exercises, or as stationary meditation."

Categories Of Qigong

"The art of qigong has three categories which are medical (or healing) Qigong, meditation qigong and martial Qigong. There are more than two thousand Qigong exercises that comprise of hundreds of different styles, engaged in moving, standing, lying or sitting. Some styles of Qigong foster Qi better than others because of their superior moves and applications – those that are simple are typically more effective and can be excellent for the central nervous system, the chronically ill, and for general health."

Meditation Qigong

"Meditation Qigong is carried out sitting, standing or lying for the purpose of mind-body integration, emotional and spiritual fulfilment, qigong cultivation and healing. It is also an effective way to relax the mind and the body. There are different types of meditation qigong, each with their own methods, techniques and objectives. Most meditation Qigong entails visualisation, focusing the qi to move to a specific part of the body, or focusing on breathing patterns, sounds, specific ideas, images and concepts. Meditation qigong is commonly applied in Chinese martial arts, while one type of meditation qigong centres on healing power to be used for oneself or others by projecting qi from the palms with the hands touching or positioned very close to the body."

What is Tai Chi?

Kellen Chia continues

"Tai chi is also a healing art that originated in China more than two thousand years ago. It is a series of continuous, circular, slow, relaxed and smooth flowing movements that has numerous health benefits for people of all ages and health conditions. Tai chi is not just a form of physical exercises; tremendous Qi is generated and circulates throughout the body when one adheres to certain theories of movement, specific posture alignment and - - in one or two of the forms- particularly breathing. The Callisthenics of Tai Chi attracts many more practitioners than Qigong, as does its feeling of fluidity of movement."

Tai Chi Forms

"The forms in Tai chi follow certain rules and involve intricate body mechanics; both are necessary conditions for the energy and power to be produced. The direction and the flow of the energy and power within the body are controlled by the forms. Done correctly, the form stimulates the energy and power, freeing up blocked pathways and allowing the qi to flow throughout the body more effectively. The aspirant needs to learn each form to a stage where it can be practised by oneself, which for a basic form can take up to twenty minutes or more depending on the form and the individual because it involves technique. The Tai Chi forms except the very simple ones – take considerably longer to learn than even the more complex forms of Qigong. And while everyone has their own natural style of movement, so long as the forms in Tai Chi comply with the specific rules the essence is retained; the forms must adhere to the Tai chi principles because otherwise the art is not Tai chi."

So there you have the main differences between Tai chi and Qigong.

To add to the above information, my friend Pauline has written a booklet about Tai chi titled "24 Forms Taiji Quan Manual" and in it she quotes a few chinese quotations:

What The Sage Says

"Even before starting the physical exercises, the state of mind is sufficient to affect the chemistry of blood circulation, vitality and metabolism."

Dr. Chu Mien Yu

'When there is no need for action, stay put. When there is no need for words, stay mute. To avoid the superfluous saves energy."

Master Liu Wei

"He who is of calm and happy nature will hardly feel the pressure of age, but to him who is of an opposite disposition youth and age are equally a burden."

Plato

In conclusion, one day as Pauline and I were deep in discussion over lunch, as we often were, I asked her how many people of her culture she knew with Cancer. She thought for a minute and said "only one that I know of"; this statement shocked me as I knew of fourteen people at the time with cancer. We asked each other, why was this so? I thought that her answer was very telling. I told her that in my opinion I thought that Asian women who keep to an oriental diet eat many leafy greens, like Chinese broccoli, bok choy, cabbage, etc. They don't drink coffee or alcohol, their drink of choice is green loose leaf tea. A brand I like is Oolong Tea which is a very superior tea, made in Taiwan, introduced to me by Pauline; and more recently she introduced me to medicinal powdered turmeric, which I take ¼ teas. dissolved in warm water most evenings, which is good to strengthen the immune system, among other things

Most traditional chinese people also don't eat bread, and then she told me their digestive systems are not designed to tolerate any dairy products. If they eat any dairy foods they feel quite sick and bloated. Some food experts say that soy products which contain phytoestrogens give Chinese women them protection from cancer, especially breast cancer, but in my opinion I think it is the many leafy greens they eat daily, as well as not eating dairy, along with plenty of ginger and garlic and drinking good quality green tea rather than regular tea or coffee.

Healthy Asian women also don't consume the amount of cakes and sweets that western women and men consume. But if Asian born people or Australian or western born Chinese switch to the western diet in a big way, they seem to get all the same deadly diseases so rife in the west like diabetes, heart attacks, cancer, arthritis, etc. In view of all this, I think there IS a significant correlation between diet and cancer.

Chapter 10

Understanding How Our Intestines Work. Fibre And Proper Bowel Motions Are The Key To Good Health

Some people may find this chapter confronting. I, however make no apologies for I think it is time for people to know what is happening to their bodies and in their digestive system and it is now time to get down to the nitty gritty. FIBRE is the key or rather LACK of it in most peoples' diets. What is actually fibre? Fibre is mostly fruits and vegetables, but in my opinion, fibre is also drinking adequate amounts of the correct fluids that aid fibre to work efficiently in one's body.

If people think they can just eat abundant amounts of fibre but neglect their fluid intake, they are deluding themselves if they think they are healthy. It is vital to drink the correct amout of fluids, that is 6-8 glasses of filtered water daily, plus juices, green or herbal tea, etc. This amount of fluids are the key to help push all the rubbish from our colons. Many people find discussing their bowel habits sickening and disgusting. Talking about the subject of bodily functions can be a turn-off for most people. It is a subject that most people find uncomfortable discussing, and is not exactly dinner party conversation, but IRONICALLY it is THE subject that we should address and discuss, if not to friends but within the family, just being aware what is and what is not a good bowel motion, and a subject doctor SHOULD talk to their patients about, if they only had the proper training on Bowel Health.

GUT health is very important and grossly overlooked by the Medical Profession. Many naturopaths trained in digestive issues refer to the Gut as the "second brain".and the brain cannot function if there is constipation present and not addressed. There is a condition known as "foggy or fuzzy brain" which means not being clear-headed, or able to focus, or short-term memory loss can occur, resulting from unchecked and long-standing constipation.

A TOXIC SYSTEM CAN CAUSE PSYCHOLOGICAL ILLNESS

According to some alternative sections of the Medical Profession it is becoming more and more apparent that an untreated toxic or constipated digestive system can cause psychological illness and disruptive thoughts and actions, which sadly can cause harm to other people.

The intestines are the sewer system of the body and most people eat and drink all the foods they like, without a thought of how or when they come out the other end. We all have about eight metres of bowel in our bodies in which is capable of storing toxins therein, that is un-expelled faecal, stagnant waste accumulating on the walls of the intestines, due to lack of fibre in our diets, and we are subconsciously self-poisoning ourselves with this faecal matter building up in the tissues. We just keep on eating and drinking everything we want without a thought of how and when it comes out at the other end, with our decadent diets and lifestyles that are putting our lives at risk, and the consequences of this is that we are literally choking in our own waste, which can and does cause serious illnesses.

When talking to people about their bowel motions, they dismiss the subject and say" oh, I don't have any trouble in that department, I go every day" or" "that's a disgusting subject - don't talk about bowel motions". When the average person goes to the bathroom to have a bowel motion, it is something that they want to get over with in a hurry and move on with their day, not bothering to take a look at their bowel motions and without a care of what they look like or how they are formed.

WHAT DEFINES A GOOD POO?

But what should bowel movements look like? A good bowel motion is when a substantial amount (enough to cover the water in the toilet bowl) of well- formed sometimes s-shaped bulky stools that look like small or large shaped tubes or bananas and "float" in the toilet bowl, not sink. One should aim to have at least one or two good bowel movements per day. Most times one bowel motion is not adequate, as some faecal matter is left behind each day and reabsorbed into the body, which is called auto-intoxication. Just having one motion a day on most days, that irregularity in itself can cause constipation and a backlog of toxins. There are different kinds of bowel motions; there are the small pellet like poos, almost diarrhoea like (not good ones) which indicate the bowels haven't been evacuated adequately and not enough fibre has been consumed the day before.

If this situation happens on a regular basis, it could be a condition called Irritable Bowel Syndrome (IBS) where people have many bowel motions a day but they are diarrhoea like, not normal or properly-formed bowel motions. Other bowel conditions are Leaky Gut syndrome and Ulcerative Colitis, conditions that can be aided with proper dietary holistic advice. There are also bowel motions that sink to the bottom of the toilet bowl so you can't even see they what they look like and when the toilet is flushed there is mostly a lot of water not faecal matter. These type of motions on a regular basis indicate constipation or build-up of toxins. These bowel motions are not desirable either, which also indicate that not enough fibre has been eaten the day before. The above bowel motions also indicate that there is bad or unfriendly bacteria in the digestive tract caused by an unhealthy diet, which could be by consuming too many carbohydrates, and/or sugary or take-away and processed foods, or by eating too much animal protein or dairy, or drinking too many cups of coffee, and/or by not eating enough fruit and vegetables and consuming soft drinks or sugary fruit juices, and also by not drinking enough water and the correct fluids. This waste matter gets left behind, adhering to the walls of the intestines; all caused by a LACK of fibre and by not drinking proper filtered drinking water and other recommended fluids to help flush out the system of excess waste matter. Healthy bowel motions are usually bulky, and those which are solidified, in large numbers and float.

There are also people who have difficulty in passing stools which get left behind in the intestines. Many people have this struggle on a daily basis or most mornings, and in often cases end up with painful haemorrhoids from straining in trying to have a good bowel motion resulting in difficult to pass stools, often having to resort to laxatives, healing creams or even more serious surgery to repair haemorrhoids.

CONSTIPATION CAN DISRUPT LIVES

This painful and time-consuming routine causes constipation and frustration, disrupting their days and can be very annoying resulting in people subconsciously start to STORE and accumulate a backlog of hard faecal waste matter, which builds up in the intestines. It may seem strange to some people but the eight or nine metres of intestines in our digestive tract are able to "store" such waste matter. Many people are oblivious to the fact that this accumulation can set themselves up for serious illnesses in the future.

There are other poos that are desirable – they are the dark bulky, almost black motions, offensive and very foul and stale smelling; these indicate constipation and old stagnant waste matter is getting removed, which can be a good sign. This old stale faecal matter has been sitting on the walls of the intestines for a long time – trapped waste which can be sitting in the colon for sometimes years, rotting and toxifying the digestive system with encrusted faecal matter not moving or budging, waiting to be expelled. This indicates true constipation and is sometimes hard to remove.

Symptoms arising out of this can be a constant feeling of bloatedness, and feeling uncomfortable, sometimes accompanied with pain in the abdominal area, and not being able to button up one's slacks or trousers, also resulting in an expanding waistline, better known as "middle-aged spread". This stagnation can start from childhood building and accumulating on the walls of the intestines.

Many health researchers have reached the conclusion that cancer cells can grow and multiply from living with years of toxic waste. The longer this toxic state remains unchecked, rotting and stagnating and injurious to health, people will find themselves with many ailments, some minor and some very serious like many forms of arthritis, diabetes, and others life threatening, like cancer, and other deadly diseases.

It is a sad fact but true that we are totally unaware of what is taking place in our bodies and the dangerous health consequences that can manifest themselves in the future, because of our toxic digestive systems. The consequences of this is called "auto-intoxication" where poisons from the intestines are re-absorbed into the bloodstream. The key to better bowel motions can be achieved by flooding the body with friendly bacteria, rather than unfriendly bacteria. Friendly bacteria can be achieved by eating lots of fibre (fruit and vegetables) by taking good quality probiotics, and following proper food combining principles. Unfriendly bacteria is when people also eat too much meat, or junk and take away food and processed food on a regular basis, and not eating enough fibre and correct fluids, therefore causing constipation and then paving the way to serious illnesses, so therefore the key to disease-free good health is to concentrate and focus on the health of the intestines.

Some patients are often prescribed antibiotics for treatment of different illnesses, but they do very little in alleviating their health issues, in many instances antibiotics only exacerbate the symptoms of their illnesses and add toxicity to their already overloaded digestive systems. It is advisable to consult with a holistic health professional who has been specifically trained to deal with intestinal conditions.

Many doctors do NOT think it is important to have a bowel motion daily and it is something that is often overlooked by them. This line of outdated thinking is how doctors are trained at Medical School. Maybe text books need to be rewritten so medical students are up-to-date with all areas of digestive health? There needs to be more bowel health education for medical students so when they complete and obtain their Medical Degrees they can pass on this knowledge to their patients, and in doing so can help to save lives!

PEOPLE ARE NOT DRINKING ENOUGH FLUIDS

To reiterate the above fluid intake recommendations, it is very important to drink adequate amounts of filtered water and healthy cleansing fruit and vegetable juice, green teas and herbal teas, as these help to flush out poisonous toxins that reside in the bowel. People should try to drink 6-8 glasses of pure water per day plus other healthy drinks as stated above (tea and coffee do not count) Sorry!

Laxatives Are Big Business

Laxatives are big business for the Pharmaceutical companies and people have created for themselves an over-dependency on them in most western countries with Americans spending a staggering $700 million annually on laxatives and the rest of the world spending another $200million annually. Yes, that adds up to $900 million annually! Shocking, isn't it?

When most people feel they are constipated they usually resort to laxatives in their many forms which when taken regularly create a dependency on them, consequently making bowels LAZY and stomach muscles FORGET how to function naturally.

Many doctors often recommend pharmaceutical laxative preparations to their patients for constipation, rather than a healthy diet, or to advise drinking more water and fluids, which would be more beneficial and a long term solution rather than a quick fix.

It is very easy for people to take laxatives thinking they can eat all the food they want and when they are bound up then take pharmaceutical laxatives or a "magic pill to get their bowels functioning. Just think, if everyone made an effort to eat healthily, we wouldn't need to spend so much money on laxatives, thus saving millions of dollars in the process, all over the world, and lessening the burden on the health system, not to mention how well we would feel! When our bowel motions are regular, it gives us a feeling of well-being and it is a good start to our day which can set the tone if we are going to have a good day or a bad day.

Colonics Helpful For Constipation
WHAT IS COLONIC LAVAGE THERAPY?

Colonic treatments can be helpful for constipation. At one stage, a couple of years ago (post cancer) I was feeling rather unwell and fatigued and rather bloated, and after an examination by the staff of The Sydney Colonic Health Clinic it was recommended to me that I needed and should have several colonic treatments as there was a faecal build-up in my intestines. Colonic treatments help to flush out waste matter in these instances. After undergoing the recommended treatments I felt much better.

Below are several passages from the Advertising Brochure of the Sydney Colon Health Clinic, explained in detail, by Bianca James, owner and founder of the above clinic.

"Colonic Lavage Therapy is a more complete and gentle form of an anaema and cleanses the entire bowel (large intestine) from rectum to caecum, detoxifying the body and providing a healthier environment for "friendly" bacteria to grow and re-colonise".

"The therapy takes around 45 minutes. Ultra purified body temperature water is slowly and gently introduced into the rectum, via a pencil-thin sterile, disposable tube."

"You are in total control of the amount of water taken in, and can eliminate into a toilet bowl built into the treatment unit whenever you feel the need."

All rooms have private facilities. Your privacy, dignity and comfort are always observed"

The Sydney Colon Health Clinic, is located at Ground floor, 50 Nicholson Street, ST. LEONARDS. N.S.W. Bianca James, operates very clean, hygienic premises, with experienced and professional staff, herself included.

Bianca James states" the bowel is the most important and the most neglected organ in the human body – keeping it working efficiently and free from toxic build-up is essential to health, healing and wellbeing"

"Problems resulting from years of improper bowel movements, poor nutrition and lifestyle cannot be resolved in a few treatments. More treatments may be required in cases of chronic constipation, irritable bowel syndrome, or auto-intoxication of the body. Probiotics – to recolonise the bowel with friendly bacteria is always recommended".

" A WORD OF CAUTION:
Colonic Lavage Therapy from Bianca James: (the medical term of the procedure) is covered under the Skin Penetration Act, 2000 and is recognised as an invasive medical procedure that should only be supervised or provided by a Registered Nurse. Unfortunately NSW Health has NOT deemed it necessary to regulate this industry, which means that anyone from any walk of life can open and operate a colonic facility and give colonics. This makes it a very dangerous procedure, as many performing colonics have no Medical qualifications, and know little if anything about Infection control. There have been reports made to the HCCC regarding unsafe practice, and they are aware of at least 6 people contracting Hep.C from visiting a clinic where, due to lack of knowledge of adequate infection Control has not been followed".

From time to time it may be necessary to have ongoing colonic irrigation treatments as toxins can recur and accumulate in the intestines, causing further constipation caused by continued faulty diet, and lack of correct fluids, resulting in discomfort, bloating and pain in the abdominal area, which sometimes causes weight gain and obesity.

From my own observations and apparently from what I have been told, there are some clinics which use instruments which can perforate the bowel, so therefore it is important to do research before embarking on any colonics treatments.

DINING OUT CAN BE PROBLEMATIC

Dining out regularly and even holidays can contribute to an overloaded digestive system because of the diet being different and eating more easy-style convenience and take away meals whilst away, different to what is normally eaten at home, with extra alcohol and extra treats consumed. This temporary change of diet and lifestyle can sometimes require a few colonic treatments. Probiotics are often recommended during and after treatments which give relief and are very helpful.

IRRITABLE BOWEL SYNDROME CAN BE RELIEVED

Irritable Bowel Syndrome sometimes called IBS often happens after a short or long bout of constipation or a change in bowel motions which can be too soft and watery or the pebble variety. Bowel motions should be solid and here again as mentioned above motions should float. IBS is a stubborn and often difficult complaint to fix, some people have the condition for ten years or more, but the condition can also be helped with colonic treatments and by feeding the body friendly bacteria, that is lots of fibre and fluids. I, myself, suffered from this ailment for a short time, but cured the condition also in a relatively short time with a few colonic treatments and by adding extra fibre to the diet, that is fruits and vegetables. (good bacteria).

CONSTIPATION – ONE OF THE CAUSES OF RECURRING HEADACHES

Constipation can cause long-standing and recurring headaches, especially in women who suffer debilitating headaches or more severe, migraines, which often force people to go to bed and lie down because of their severity, until the pain subsides. Only a sufferer knows just how bad these headaches can be. Sufferers often have to resort to pain killers or stronger medications such as analgesics. These medications can be expensive if used on a regular basis, but only serve as a temporary relief and actually do very little in alleviating their pain permanently and getting to the bottom of the cause and therefore medications are "bandaid" solutions.

Alternatively, when headaches are addressed through eating a healthy diet and detoxifying the digestive tract of years of toxic waste, many headache sufferers report that the headaches that caused lifelong misery and pain no longer exist. By adopting detoxifying measures and ridding the body of unwanted waste can give people a much clearer head thus relieving their headaches.

Admittedly, there are other reasons for headaches like eyestrain or misaligned neck problems or other unexplained reasons, which should be checked out, BUT

I CURED MY OWN HEADACHES

I, myself am a testimony for treating headaches with a change of diet as I once suffered shocking headaches and often times when I suffered migraines regularly, which were almost every week which also forced me to lie down in a darkened room away from glaring light and noise. I now no longer suffer with headaches and have not had an episode for many years. If I do rarely get a headache it is usually very mild and does not last long, which proves that I am a testimony for treating headaches naturally, through corrective diet, without any medication.

Chapter 11

Breast Cancer Is On The Increase

Breast Cancer is frighteningly on the increase in western countries and in Australia 15000 women each year will be diagnosed with breast cancer in Australia. How many of these women will survive long term? How many of these women will survive the magic 5 year survival rate and beyond?

Bernard Jensen, D.C., Ph.D.,ND Nutritionist, born way ahead of his time writes about the link between constipation and breast cancer – below is a passage taken from one of Bernard Jensen's books titled "Tissue cleansing through bowel Management" co-authored with Sylvia Bell, 1981 12th edition.

The following clipping is from the Daily News Service, 1981:

CANCER RISK FOR WOMEN

"A new study by University of San Francisco medical researchers has revived turn–of–the–century idea that toxic substances produced in the bowel can have damaging health effects. The study's findings also support recent suggestions of a link between a diet high in fat and low in fibre and an increased risk of developing breast cancer. The study of 1,481 non-nursing women showed that those who are severely constipated tend to have abnormal cells in the fluid extracted from their breasts. Such cells have been found in

women with breast cancer and, the researchers suggested, may indicate that the women face an increased risk of developing cancer. The cellular abnormalities occurred five times as often in women who moved their bowels fewer than three times a week than in women who did so more than once a day. Chronic constipation is often the result of a diet high in protein, fat and refined carbo-hydrates (sugars and refined flour) but low in such fibrous foods such as whole grains, fruit and vegetables".

Very telling indeed! It is becoming clearer to me that if the above passage is correct and constipation and breast cancer are linked, it would be reasonable to suggest that many other types of cancer may also be linked to constipation (toxaemia). More information on Dr Bernard Jensen below.

OBESITY IS ON THE INCREASE

Fifty years ago obesity was almost an unknown and rarely used word to describe overweight and obese people who were in the minority. Today it is a very different story, the reverse is true.

With 63% of Australians and Americans now being overweight or obese, you can't help noticing their bulging bellies and large backsides. One reason is a change in the very different diet from fifty years ago, compared to today's diet and lifestyle. Fifty years ago people stayed at home more and prepared home-cooked meals and got more exercise in their daily lives.

Today many people lead sedentary lifestyles working in front of computers and a reliance and focus on eating take-away foods and dining out at restaurants on a regular basis. One reason for this dining trend is there are two or more incomes in a family and there is more disposable income. In some cases people have become more affluent. A sad consequence of this is overweight and obesity. The reason then for all men with the "beer belly gut" and middle-age spread" and layers of "spare tyres" in women is that they are carrying around a lot of waste matter in their intestines and many of them are constipated but are not aware of it (belly fat) The overloaded intestines have nowhere to go so consequently peoples' abdomens are pushed forward with the heavy overload of putrefying faecal matter in their intestines.

For those people who are overweight or obese, a good detoxifying diet will aid in losing weight, which includes lots of fresh fruit and vegetables, drinking filtered water, eating less junk food and sweets, cakes and biscuits, cutting back on coffee and less reliance on take away and processed foods. These measures will help them to lose those unwanted kilos, and help maintain a healthy body weight, by detoxifying their digestive systems, giving them better bowel motions, consequently lightening the load on the intestines and ridding the body of cancer-causing toxins and possibly other serious diseases.

People who address the diet with the above measures can go a long way to PREVENT serious illness from starting in the first place. There is an old saying that goes like this: "an ounce of prevention is better than a ton of cure".

Detoxifying The System – Makes Weight Loss Easier

I find that when the bowels are addressed and adopt a vegetarian or a semi-vegetarian diet with lots of filtered water and plenty of salads and fruit and vegetables, by detoxifying the system, takes the burden and weight off the intestines, it is possible to maintain a healthy body weight. Continuing to detoxify the digestive tract also helps to achieve that elusive flat stomach that we all desire to have.

Exercise is important too, but you don't have to SWEAT IT OUT at the gym. Heavy physical exercise and gym work alone will NOT shift the weight if you are NOT on a diet that detoxifies the digestive system. All the exercise in the world, or sweating it out in saunas or gyms or excessively long walks or other forms of exercise alone cannot or will not shift weight, if people are not on healthy diets!

If people are overweight or obese, health professionals should be consulted before embarking on any form of exercise.

How Do We Know If We Have High Levels Of Toxicity?

Below is a list of just some of the symptoms of toxicity:

1. Excessive and foul smelling flatulence.
2. Abdominal bloating.
3. Coated tongue and bad breath.
4. Lack of energy accompanied with constant tiredness and to a greater extent chronic fatigue syndrome, and being overweight or obese.
5. Anaemia
6. Pasty looking skin
7. Regular colds and bronchitis and bouts of flu and cold sores or mouth ulcers or irritations
8. Regular headaches which can be mild or in extreme cases unrelenting severe migraines
9. Arthritis ranging from mild to severity can be involved in some instances.
10. Skin irritations, a relentless itchy scalp or more severe cases of psoriasis of the scalp or other parts of the body.

Incontinence And Back Pain Can Be Linked To Toxins

Many women today suffer from incontinence which can be very embarrassing. There are different schools of thought as to what causes this frustrating and lingering ailment, one symptom is frequency of urinating. Many years ago I had occasion to consult a naturopath who specialised in bowel problems and constipation. She showed me an x-ray of a woman's intestines, which visibly showed the bursting heavy weight of the intestines overloaded with faecal matter creating pressure and prolapse of the bladder consequently causing incontinence.

Prolapse of the bladder can also be caused by the pelvic muscles of the bladder which have been stretched from childbirth causing the bladder to descend down into the vagina causing incontinence. It can be especially common in menopausal, overweight or obese women.

Similarly, cases of slight or severe back pain can be caused by an overload of toxins in the bowel, pressing on the lower discs of the spine and vertebrae, causing the discs to swell and bulge, creating much pain and discomfort in the lower back.

In these instances this is where learning to detoxify the body of trapped waste can help to eliminate incontinence and back pain. Sometimes unsuspecting doctors may recommend back and bladder operations which may not be necessary.

Maybe the treatment could be as simple as addressing the intestines so reducing the need for painful, costly and unnecessary operations which aren't always successful, sometimes the condition returns because the toxic state of the intestines has not been addressed and further unnecessary operations may be prescribed by some medical professionals.. There are however occasions when operations may be absolutely necessary for people with constant chronic back pain.

Before considering any operations for prolapse, there is an informative article written on Female bladder and uterine prolapse by Lyn Craven, who is a practitioner of naturopathy and Bowen therapy, meditation teacher, health writer and corporate health facilitator, the article is "Natural Therapies for Prolapse, Part 2" Her website is:

www.lyncravencorporatehealth-naturopath.com.

Chapter 12

Tips To Get The Bowels Moving

Cleansing of the intestines should be done in the morning. A certain time should be set aside a to kick-start the bowels, that is first thing in the morning which is the best time to evacuate the bowels on an empty stomach, and when I say detoxify I don't mean a harsh purging, diarrhoea kind of inner cleansing, but bowel motions should come our rather easily with just a slight push, no straining.

One of my tips to get the bowels moving is to have 2 large glasses (200mls) of warm filtered water (not tap water) with a SMALL squeeze of lemon, one after the other; lemon juice contains enzymes that stimulate the liver, and lemon juice helps to cleanse the bowel flushing out waste matter more efficiently and stimulates and releases gastric juices getting the bowels to move less effortlessly, without straining, (provided healthy eating has taken place the day before). Why drink warm water? It is important to drink the lemon water warm rather than cold water as drinking cold water only goes straight to the stomach; warm water goes straight to the intestines, and acts like an anaema, loosening and softening faecal matter for easier expulsion. I find room temperature can be cold also, especially in winter, so it is advisable to heat the water slightly as it tastes more palatable and easier to get down, sending an urgent message to the intestines to have a bowel motion, then shifting the old faecal matter that sits on the intestinal walls, After a second bowel motion, (hopefully) it is important to then have a vegetable and fruit juice. (recipe in a later chapter) Now here is the important trick – (a tip one of my children stumbled upon), you press your stomach or lean against your kitchen bench and wait for a few minutes; this pressure on the stomach muscles, sends a message to the organs of elimination, namely the liver, the kidneys through the urine, think good kidney health by all the fluids recommended above, to flush the kidneys out and finally the intestinal muscles are stimulated giving the urge to go to the bathroom for bowel evacuation. This procedure usually works provided the correct fibre has been eaten the day before. Whilst waiting for this urge to use your bowels, you can do a crossword or some reading matter, which helps to relax the body and mind. This process may take several minutes.

In order to obtain the second bowel motion, whilst still pressing the abdomen against the kitchen bench, you should eat a large serve of watermelon and a serve of granny smith apple or soft pear (skin on) I then have a THIRD glass warm water with lemon and by this time the second bowel motion should be on its way. Sounds way out? Maybe it does, but it works for me and it should work for others too. Perseverance, determination and focus on diet are the key elements to good bowel health and overall health in general. If good bowel health is present the rest should follow. Some days it is not always possible to have two good bowel movements; this depends on what was consumed the day or days before. A change in eating habits or dining out or holidays can all influence digestion and bowel habits.

BEST TO DRINK MOST FLUID INTAKE IN THE MORNING AND THE REST LATER IN THE DAY AND EVENING

By drinking a big quota of fluids in the morning, the intestines have a better chance of working efficiently on a still rather empty stomach, rather than drinking most fluids in the afternoon or in the evening. If most fluids are drunk late in the afternoon or evening you will have to get up and go the bathroom a couple of times during the night to urinate, which can disrupt sleep.

COFFEE IS NOT RECOMMENDED EARLY MORNING

For those people who dive for their coffee pots first thing in the morning, followed by orange juice, toast and cereal, THINK AGAIN. This procedure could be detrimental to your health. Why? Because after having a long fast during sleep, it is necessary to get the intestines to work first thing in the morning with the above procedures, on an empty stomach. It is important to follow the above procedures on an empty stomach, that is drinking most of the fluids FIRST, before eating anything solid. This procedure usually results in achieving the first bowel motion of the day. People who eat food first thing in the morning, with their coffee or tea, without the proper fluids, on an empty stomach, are setting themselves up for illness and constipation, by putting more and more solid food into their bodies, without giving their intestines a chance to eliminate their already trapped waste. It then makes it harder to achieve good bowel motions, maybe then having to resort to laxatives for quick results, which is not advisable as they can create a dependency on them. If laxatives are taken regularly they will not work successfully long term. If other foods and coffee or tea are taken continuously, first thing on rising, day after day, week after week, with little or no attention to inner cleansing, faecal build-up in the intestines can result, causing discomfort, bloating and inevitable disease.

If people are time poor and working there may not be enough time for the above procedures that take up extra effort in the morning, but by rising half an hour earlier it can be achieved and it is very worthwhile to get the best results rather than waiting for the weekends only, when there is more time for such procedures. but the down side is you are possibly building up more and more waste matter in the intestines by adopting the above measures only at weekends.

When time permits, it is worthwhile persevering with the above methods, although which may seem unusual to some people, it is worth it to get maximum results with clarity of mind, and a sense of wellbeing. Proper daily cleansing of the intestines also makes it easier to maintain a healthy weight, without having to resort to drastic measures like abnormally long walks or heavy workouts at the gym, which can be costly and often don't always work.

"Death Starts In The Bowel" Bernard Jensen's Early Comments On Bowel Cleansing

"Death starts in the Bowel"

This is a phrase made famous by Dr Bernard Jensen.

According to Wikipedia, Dr. Bernard Jensen, was an early pioneer in nutrition and authority on bowel health, lived to the ripe old age of 93, his longevity a testimony in itself, attributed to the healthy way he lived as he practised what he preached. He himself suffered from a lung disease and turned to study foods that have an impact on health and wellbeing. Dr Jensen also operated several health sanitariums in California throughout his lifetime, having spent 60 years of his career successfully treating patients in his health sanitariums and health ranches. During his life he saved many peoples' lives and was recorded as having consulted 350,000 patients by teaching them the correct diet and healthy lifestyle and authored over 50 books.

According to Bernard Jensen International, Dr. Jensen's work is still carried out today by his son, Art, and daughter-in-law, Ellen, as they studied alongside the legendary natural healer, Dr. Bernard Jensen, many years before, learning from him everything he had to teach in the fields of Iridology, nutrition, cleansing, supplements and numerous other healing methods".

Read more about the Jensens on:
http://www.bernardjensen.com/About-Us- -ep 7.html

Cleansing The Colon

Dr Jensen comments on bowel cleansing:

"Researchers have found that a lack of fibre in the diet increases the transit time of bowel matter to sit in the intestines stimulating production of putrefactive bacteria in the bowel. This is what is known as auto-intoxication where poisons that should have been removed from our body via the intestines are simply reabsorbed right back into the bloodstream. Post Mortems evidence that people carry about 15-18 pounds of impacted, putrefying faecal matter in their colons".

Doctor Bernard Jensen, DC, ND, Ph.D., made the following statement. "In the 50 years I've spent helping people to overcome illness, disability and disease; it has become crystal clear that poor bowel health management lies at the root of most people's health problems."

The information about breast cancer and constipation written by Dr, Jensen in the above passages seem to have a very strong link with each other and conventional medicine may need to address these issues.

Dr. Bernard Jensen studied with many very successful doctors throughout the United States and Europe.

In his book *Tissue Cleansing Through Bowel Management*, Dr. Jensen discusses Mucoid Plaque. He writes: "The heavy mucous coating in the colon thickens and becomes a host of putrefaction. The blood capillaries to the colon begin to pick up the toxins, poisons and noxious debris as it seeps through the bowel wall. All tissues and organs of the body are now taking on toxic substances. Here is the beginning of true autointoxication on a physiological level".

"On page 42, Dr. Jensen talks about his old teacher John Harvey Kellogg at the Battle Creek Sanitarium who maintained that 90% of the diseases of civilization are due to improper functioning of the Colon. On page 27 Dr. Jensen reveals his experience in this matter. "One autopsy revealed a colon to be 9 inches in diameter with a passage through it no larger than a pencil. The rest was caked up layer upon layer of encrusted faecal material. This accumulation can have the consistency of truck tire rubber. It's that hard and black. ANOTHER AUTOPSY REVEALED A STAGNANT COLON TO WEIGH IN AT AN INCREDIBLE 40LBS. Imagine carrying around all that morbid accumulated waste".

Chapter 13

Cancer And Birth Defects In Babies And Young Children

Forty years ago cancer and birth defects in babies and young children were practically unheard of. With today's technology to make life easier and a totally different shift in lifestyles and diets, along with environmental factors, there seems to have brought about more and more occurring serious cancers and birth defects in babies and young children. Below are some of the consequences of risky lifestyles and wrongful dietary habits that can adversely affect the health of a baby in utero.

It all starts in the womb. A healthy baby is created in the womb. A healthy baby is no accident. Once a woman discovers she is pregnant it is up to her to practise good nutrition with a reasonable amount of exercise. Before embarking on starting a family, couples ought to realise the responsibility involved in taking care of a child, and it is a step to be taken very seriously, not a step to be taken lightly, therefore they should look at the state of their diets and lifestyles and if they are taking any illicit drugs or prescription drugs, smoking, etc. as these lifestyle habits can have a deleterious effect on their unborn child. However, there are times when pregnancies just happen unexpectedly, as in the case of teenage or unwanted pregnancies. There are several steps mothers and fathers-to-be can take to ensure that they produce a healthy baby. Parents-to-be may follow all the guidelines recommended in this chapter, but even with all the careful preparation things unfortunately can go wrong at the time of delivery from maybe lack of oxygen to the brain of the newborn baby or other unforeseen circumstances causing serious consequences to the newborn baby. Below are some of the things parents-to-be can do even BEFORE they decide to have a baby.

Diet And Obesity

It is a well-known fact in medical circles that overweight or obese mothers-to-be (and fathers) can have difficulty falling pregnant, so it is advisable for couples (males too) to try to lose any excess weight they may be carrying around and try to maintain a healthy weight.

THE DAILY MAIL states and web page
http//www.dailymail.co.uk/health/article-
2285627/Obese-m.. 30/10.2013

Obese Mothers 'Put Babies' Hearts At Risk: Infants Show Early Stages Of Disease When They Are Born

- Babies born to obese mothers had thicker artery walls at birth.
- A third of women of childbearing age are overweight, 20 per cent are obese

By *Jenny Hope*
PUBLISHED: 00:19 GMT, 28th February 2013
UPDATED: 01:50 GMT, 28th February 2013

"Babies whose mothers are overweight or obese show early signs of heart disease at birth, warn researchers.

"Scans of newborn infants with fat mothers found they have thicker artery walls – a sign of heart disease-than those born to women of 'normal' weight.

"The arterial thickening occurred independently of the child's weight at birth, which is a known risk factor for heart disease or stroke in later life".

"Experts from Nottingham University say the early difference detected in a major artery could explain why a mother's weight during pregnancy is so influential to their child's subsequent risk of cardiovascular problems".

"Obesity affects around 20 per cent of all women of childbearing age, with a further third being overweight".

"The latest study included 23 women, with an average age of 35, whose body Mass Index (BMI) scores ranged from being underweight to seriously obese at 16 weeks of pregnancy."

"Researchers from Sydney University, Australia, scanned the abdominal aorta- the section of the artery extending down to the belly – in each newborn within seven days of birth to find out the thickness of the two innermost walls – the intima and media".

"The latest findings add to evidence that internal fat levels in the newborn baby are directly related to the mother's weight during pregnancy".

"Scans of babies less than 12 days old by researchers at Imperial College London found a direct link between a mother's weight and the build-up in fat around their baby's abdomen in the same way as people in their 50s."

"Previous research by Nottingham University looking at data from 30 studies of 200,000 people found children born to mothers who are overweight face a higher risk of being fat themselves throughout childhood and their teens."

"Being overweight and smoking during pregnancy increase the chances still further of children being obese, along with being heavy at birth and rapid weight gain as a baby."

"Amy Thompson, Senior Cardiac Nurse at the British Heart Foundation (BHF) said "These results could suggest a direct link between a mother's weight during pregnancy and her child's risk of cardiovascular disease ."

"If you're thinking of starting a family and have concerns about your weight, try to eat healthily and keep active."

"Looking after yourself when you're pregnant will mean that you are in the best position to look after your baby when the time comes"'.

The above article can be read in full on the above web page.

Junk Food In Pregnancy Can Contribute To Many Health Issues In The Unborn Child

According to DEAKIN UNIVERSITY Australia Worldly, And written by Associate Professor Felice Jacka.

Webpage
http://www.deakin.edu.au/news/2013/200813junkfoo dmental... 28/10/2013

'JUNK FOOD MAY LEAD TO MENTAL HEALTH PROBLEMS IN CHILDREN
20th August 2013

New research suggests that mums with unhealthy diets during pregnancy are more likely to have children with behavioural problems. It has also shown that children with unhealthy diets have increased symptoms of depression and anxiety, as well as aggression and tantrums.

"Deakin University researchers, working with Norwegian collaborators, have found for the first time that a clear relationship exists between mum's diets during pregnancy, as well as children's diets during the first years of life, and children's mental health".

"We've known for quite some time that very early life nutrition, including the nutrition received while the child is in utero, is related to physical health outcomes in children – their risk for later heart disease or diabetes for example. But this is the first study indicating that diet is also important to mental health outcomes in children, "said ASSOCIATE PROFESSOR FELICE JACKA, lead author of the study and researcher with Deakin University's IMPACT Strategic Research Centre based at Barwon Health in Geelong.

"Depression and anxiety disorders account for some of the leading causes of disability worldwide. Recent research has established that diet and nutrition are related to the risk for these common mental disorders in adults and adolescents. However, no studies have examined the impact of very early life nutrition and its relationship to mental health in children, until now".

"This latest study, funded by the Brain & Behaviour Research foundation, involved more than 23,000 mothers and their children participating in the large, ongoing Norwegian Mother and Child cohort Study (Moba). The study gathered detailed information on mothers' diets during pregnancy and their children's diets at 18 months and three years."

"The results of the study, published in the Journal of the American Academy of Child and Adolescent Psychiatry, suggested that mums who eat more unhealthy foods, such as refined cereals, sweet drinks, and salty snacks, during pregnancy have children with more behavioural problems, such as tantrums and aggression. It also shows that children who eat more unhealthy foods during the first years of their life, or who do not eat enough nutrient rich foods , such as vegetables, exhibit more of these 'externalizing' behaviours indicative of depression and anxiety. These relationships were independent of other factors that may explain these links, such as the socio-economic circumstances or mental health of the parents."

Associate Professor Jacka said that as the negative impact of unhealthy foods on the waistline of our population grows, so does the evidence suggesting that our mental health is also affected.

"It is becoming clearer that diet matters to mental health right across the age spectrum," she said.

"These new findings suggest that unhealthy and 'junk' foods may have an impact on the risk for mental health problems in children and they add to the growing body of evidence on the impact of unhealthy diets on the risk for depression, anxiety and even dementia".

"The changes to our food systems, including the shift to more high-energy, low nutrition foods developed and marketed by the processed food industry, have led to a massive increase in obesity-related illnesses right across the globe."

"There is an urgent need for governments everywhere to take note of the evidence and amend food policy to restrict the marketing and availability of unhealthy food products to the community," Associate Professor Jacka said.

Lack Of Cooking Skills To-Day

One of the reasons why there are so many overweight and obese women and men (and children, of course) in western countries today is that many of today's woman have forgotten to learn to cook, or aren't very interested in the whole domestic thing, mostly due to the advent of the feminist movement which started to take hold in the 1970s after women liberated themselves from the kitchen and joined the work force. They wanted equal rights for women like their male counterparts, and many had the opportunity to go to work or study at University for their chosen careers even though they had children. Unlike many of today's young women, the women from my generation (the Baby Boomers) were happy to stay home and do all the domestic things like cooking, cleaning, dressmaking, etc. and be a home-maker. Housewives of yesteryear were from a very different upbringing and mentality. Generally girls learnt to bake cakes when they were teenagers, cooking for the family and most girls grew up in an environment where most mothers didn't work but stayed at home and made home cooked meals, so learning domestic skills for young women was a very natural thing and very empowering, thus leaving them in good stead when they eventually married and had their own children. These cooking and domestic skills, even learning how to manage housekeeping money, gave them knowledge to keep them in good stead, knowing how to cook for their husbands and children, and running a household on a budget, and also feeling confidently capable of entertaining friends and family.

Whilst the next two generations (gen X and Y) have been busy forging a corporate or professional careers (which is highly commendable I might add), they don't think cooking is as important as their careers. Cooking for them is not cool and is not an option. Maybe that is one reason why many men have taken over the role of cook and home maker whilst women are out working hard to help pay for their mortgages.

Working couples also prefer to dine out regularly or pick up a convenient take-away meal on their way home from work. Another factor for today's families eating out regularly is that with couples both working, they have more disposable income and can easily afford to dine out often at restaurants or rely on convenience or fast foods. There are also too many fast food options around today; one only have to pick up the phone and your meal will be delivered to your door, or you can go a drive through fast foot outlet, order your meal and it is delivered to your car. It is too easy in today's world to rely on takeaway and junk foods, thus making people very lazy.

HOPE FOR THE FUTURE FOR RECENT GENERATIONS

It is desirable and remains to be seen if Gen. Z (those born from 1995-2015) will bring back a revival of cooking skills for women (and men) and Generations

X and Y find a new "awakening" for cooking, combined with a desire for domesticity, especially in the kitchen, making cooking "cool" again. Baby Boomers and those slightly younger would remember the days when cooking classes, better known as "Home Science" classes were automatically included in the schools' curriculum, but these classes were only provided at certain schools. Home Science classes seemed to disappear during the period cooking was considered "uncool" and these courses were replaced with more important and relevant subjects like Asian and other languages and computer technology classes, forcing cooking classes out of the equation.

On the positive side I believe cooking classes in schools are reappearing on the scene, due to the rising demand probably spurred on by the influx of cooking shows on TV and competition TV shows over the last few years, with children also wanting to take part in these shows, whilst cooking gourmet meals at home for their families, many of them as young as 10 and 11 yr. olds. There are also many more cook books appearing these days, which adorn the shelves of book stores everywhere; these cook-books, containing countless interesting recipes from many different cultures.

Cigarette Smoking Is Implicated With Birth Defects On New-Borns And Young Children

There is good documented evidence that cigarette smoking can have devastating effects on the unborn child, causing cancer to develop in babies, if not immediately after birth, but later on in early childhood. Doctors and nurses in pre-natal classes are advising women to give up smoking whilst pregnant. There is also evidence that babies can be born with physical defects as well as mental abnormalities, with mothers to be, or more importantly by the father-to-be who is also a smoker, light or heavy; smoking can adversely affect the sperm. ANY smoking is too much smoking. MEN ALSO need to take a good look at their smoking habits, diet and lifestyle before starting a family. The quality of a man's sperm is often overlooked but is an important factor when couples are planning to start a family.

It has also been documented that babies who are exposed to second-hand smoke before and after birth have a very high risk for SIDS (sudden infant death syndrome) than babies whose parents do NOT SMOKE or have exposure to second-hand smoke.

Childhood Cancers
Are Common

What Is Neuroblastoma?

According to the Children's Neuroblastoma Cancer Foundation, it is the third most common type of childhood cancer after leukaemia and brain tumours. Neuroblastoma is a solid tumour cancer of the sympathetic nervous system that originates in the nerve tissue of the neck, chest, abdomen, or pelvis, but most commonly in the adrenal gland. The average age of children diagnosed with neuroblastoma is 22 months.

Signs And Symptoms
Of Neuroblastoma

- A swollen stomach, abdominal pain and decreased appetite (if the tumour is in the abdomen.
- Bone pain or soreness, black eyes, bruises, and pale skin (if the cancer has spread to the bones).
- Weakness, numbness, inability to move a body part, or difficulty walking (if the cancer presses on the spinal cord).
- Drooping eyelid, unequal pupils, sweating, and red skin, which are signs of nerve damage in the neck known as Horner's syndrome (if the tumour is in the neck).

- Difficulty breathing (if the cancer is in the chest).

The Childrens' Neuroblastoma Cancer Foundation continues:

"Neuroblastoma, once unheard of is now responsible for 15% of all childhood deaths in Australia each year and damage can develop in the uterus. According to the Children's Cancer Institute of Australia, 40 children each year are diagnosed in Australia with Neuroblastoma alone. 700 children are diagnosed each year in the US with Neuroblastoma. Lymphoblastoma is another common cancer diagnosed in babies and young children today. More staggeringly, statistics show that approximately 156 babies and young children die from all cancers each year in Australia and approx. 1545 babies and young children die each year in the US, and these numbers are rising. Any deaths from childhood cancers are too many and very tragic."

"Although rates of survival are improving in babies and young children, survivors of childhood cancers are a risk of developing at least one medical disability or problem as a direct result of their medical therapies. Cancer treatments like chemotherapy and radiation can cause long term side effects so children who survive cancer need careful attention for the rest of their lives."

The information on Neuroblastoma can be read in full at:

http://kidshealth/org/parent/medical/cancer/neuroblastoma. html/2/4/2013

Male Sperm Count
At An All Time Low

"Documented data shows males' sperm counts are at an all time low. One in five men aged between 18 and 25 produce abnormal sperm counts of poor quality. Professor Skakkeback from the University of Copenhagen presented data indicating sperm counts had fallen by about a half over the past fifty years."

Valuation information is available on line from ASH, an Australian Public Charity Organisation authority on tobacco smoking and its consequences on the unborn baby.

Go to
http:.www.ahaust.org//LV/
LV3informationparents.htm.

According to a publication from ASH, states "PREGNANT SMOKE EXPOSURE HARMS BABIES' BRAIN DEVELOPMENT 2012: A study of 282 newborns shows not just active smoking but second-hand exposure during pregnancy can harm various features of babies' brain development – regardless of socio-economic or medical variables"

"MATERNAL SMOKING MAY MULTIPLY CHILD BRAIN TUMOUR RISK March 2013: An Australian study of over 300 cases (900 controls) of childhood brain tumour shows five times higher incidence in young children whose mothers smoke before or during pregnancy. Authors caution about study's "modest numbers" call for more research"

Abstract

Children Of Smoking Dads More Likely To Develop Leukaemia 2011: "Children whose fathers smoked at time of conception have 15% higher risk of developing acute lymphoblastic leukaemia – the most common childhood cancer. Australian-led study compared data from 300 children with leukaemia to 800 without." Daily Mail 15/12/11

Tobacco Industry Still Targeting Children – And How To Fight It: Us Surgeon-General 2012: "Report from the US Surgeon-General finds: Tobacco industry promotion is still hooking children into smoking: and comprehensive strategies including tax, public education and smoke free policies are helping reduce youth smoking and uptake" Report

Tobacco Industry Using New Media To Reach Young Audience 2011: "Sydney University study shows tobacco companies using social media networks to reach young targets. Author suggests need to re-examine tobacco control to close this promotional loophole. Abstract.

For more valuable information on the effects of cigarette smoking and its consequences, I recommend reading the literature published from the ASH

Organisation which is available on line. Go to the web page,

http://www.ashaust.org.au//lv3/Lv3informationpare
nts.htm 2/04/2013

As you will read in the following passages fathers-to-be do not get off the hook in creating a baby; to the contrary, the male partner's diet and lifestyle is JUST as important as the diet and lifestyle of the mother-to-be.

Fathers-To-Be Need To Be Attentive

Smoking Fathers

THE CONVERSATION MEDIA GROUP writes:
"HEY DAD, YOUR HEALTH AFFECTS YOUR BABY'S WELL-BEING TOO taken from the website:

http://theconversation.com/hey-dad-your-health-
affects-your-... 18/04/2013

According to The Conversation Media Group " and David Gardner, Head of the Department of Zoology at University of Melbourne along with Dr Natalie Hannan NHMRC Early Career Research Fellow at University of Melbourne and PhD student Natalie binder write "Almost 20% of Australian adult males smoke despite its well-publicised health risks. Studies from China, Australia and Europe have identified an approximately 30% increase in the rate of childhood cancers when fathers smoke prior to conception. As a society, we put a significant emphasis on women's health both immediately prior to and during pregnancy – and rightly so. A woman needs to prepare her body for the arduous nine months of gestation ahead to give the growing baby the best possible start to life".

"A pregnant woman is likely to take supplements and maintain a healthy diet free of alcohol and cigarettes while protecting herself from unnecessary environmental toxin exposure. In comparison, men's health prior to conception is relatively insignificant right? WRONG!"

Enter Father

"Our research shows that male diet prior to conception – particularly a fast-food-based-diet can be significantly detrimental to pregnancy success. Using an animal model of diet-induced obesity, we compared pregnancy outcomes when fathers were either normal weight or obese. We found that rates of pregnancy were significantly lower when the father was obese because embryos generated with sperm from obese males weren't very good and failed to implant into the mother's uterus."

"When obese fathers were able to achieve a pregnancy, the resulting foetus and placenta were both smaller than normal and the foetus was developmentally delayed. As the theory of the developmental origins of health and disease suggests, these small-for-gestational-age foetus are at a higher risk of disease in later life, including cardiovascular disease, type 2 diabetes and high blood pressure."

"Indeed, our data indicate that being an obese male could significantly compromise the health of the resultant offspring. Initial studies in humans have also shown that the time taken to become pregnant is significantly longer if the father is obese, and IVF embryos are of poorer quality".

"This is of particular concern given the rising rates of global obesity."

Smoking Fathers Also A Risk To The Unborn Child

"And bad diet isn't the only vice of modern man that can affect not only fertility but also the health of his offspring. Almost 20% of Australian adult males smoke despite its well-publicised health risks. Studies from China, Australia and Europe have identified an approximately 30% increase in the rate of childhood cancers when fathers smoke prior to conception".

"In particular, the rate of leukaemia, lymphoma and brain tumours were up to 80% higher in children under the age of five when FATHERS had smoked prior to conception, even though mothers were non-smokers. And the rate of childhood cancer was highest when fathers smoked more cigarettes per day, had been smoking for a longer time, and started smoking before the age of 20".

What's more, passive smoke exposure of mothers around the time of conception – likely due to fathers' smoking – is associated with a significantly high incidence off serious congenital heart defects in infants."

The Dangers Of Work

"While the effects of paternal diet, smoking, and alcohol consumption on offspring health can be mitigated with appropriate lifestyle changes before starting a family, occupational toxin exposure is harder to avoid".

"A recent study involving almost 10,000 children with birth defects was able to relate the rate of foetal malformation to job types their fathers did. Overwhelmingly, fathers exposed to solvents and chemicals in the workplace, such as artists, cleaners, hairdressers, scientists, welders, metal and food processing workers have significantly higher rates of a variety of birth defects among their offspring."

Passing It On

"Damage or changes to the male line germ line, the sperm, is how paternal lifestyle and occupation end up having a detrimental effect on foetal development and offspring health. Sperm are particularly vulnerable to oxidative stress, which can damage DNA. And both a high-fat diet and smoking have been associated with increasing levels of oxidative stress."

"Fathers' health prior to conception is clearly just as important as mothers' and when thinking of starting a family both mum and dad need to be as healthy as possible."

Other Groups At Risk In Certain Industries In The Workplace

THE EUROPEAN AGENCY FOR SAFETY & HEALTH AT WORK (OSHWIKI) states:

"Other occupations that can be responsible for birth defects where there are chemicals used are shoemakers, the printing industry, the metal industry, painters, spray painting on cars and the smash repairing industry, panel beaters, degreasing, shoe makers, the dry cleaning industry, the cleaning industry and its products, hospital workers and the pharmaceutical industry, furniture makers and cabinet makers, etc."

If people become aware what jobs and chemicals are harmful to themselves and that cause birth defects to the unborn child, it may be possible to be moved to sections of that particular organisation where maybe there are fewer dangerous chemicals to be inhaled or wear protective clothing, or change their jobs completely, if that option is possible or desirable.

Parents-to-be who are embarking on starting a family should first be made aware of all the chemical solvents lurking in the workplace and around the home, in that they can subconsciously be inhaling dangerous chemicals every day, day after day, oblivious to the possible health hazards to their own health and that of their unborn child, resulting in birth defects or even cancer. Whilst parents-to-be think they are having a healthy lifestyle with correct diet and exercise, they may be unaware of the many different types of chemical solvents surrounding them in their workplaces and homes.

Parenting a child can be a stressful experience at the best of times, but when giving birth to a child with severe or even mild defects, this situation can impact on the parents' lives in such a way which they never would have expected in that it is an unforeseen, stressful, worrying and difficult period for the parents with some of their child's defects being long term and no cure.

For more information on the above and a list of many of the occupations at risk for birth defects and cancer go to the above website.

Warning – BPA – Free Plastic Containers May Be Just As Hazardous

Warns *Dr. J. Mercola*
Retrieved DEC. 10TH, 2014.

Dr. Joseph Mercola, an American health expert, and an alternative proponent and osteopathic physician and a web entrepreneur and The New York Times best-selling author with his insight on a variety of health issues and has been interviewed on CNN, The Today Show, ABC World News, Dr. Oz show, the Doctors, Time Magazine and Forbes, according to Wikipedia. Dr. Mercola writes:

"Plastic chemicals can and do leach from plastic containers, thereby contaminating food and beverages. In the past, plastic was thought as an inert substance. Now we know that plastic chemicals can and do leach from plastic containers, thereby contaminating the foods and beverages they hold. Among the most hazardous of these chemicals known to date are bisphenol –A (BPA) and phthalates, both of which mimic hormones in your body. Even tiny concentrations can cause problems, and you're likely being exposed from a wide variety of sources."

"Aside from canned goods, they're found in reusable food containers, plastic wraps, water bottles, personal care products – you name it. In response to consumer demand for BPA –free products, many manufacturers have switched to using a different chemical called bisphenol – S (BPS). Alas, BPS appears to be just as toxic. Endocrine disrupting chemicals can affect sexual development – fertility."

"Environmental toxins from BPAs and BPS can be responsible for serious health conditions such as cancers, autism disorder, heart disease and mental conditions.

"As I see it people who are the most vulnerable to being exposed to chemicals in BPAS AND BPS and Phthalates are babies, pregnant women and women in general, followed by the rest of the population.

"Ovarian toxicity appears to be a particularly strong feature of BPA. Harvard researchers have found that higher BPA levels in women are linked to a reduced number of fertile eggs."

The rest of Dr. Mercola's article on the subject of Endocrine Disrupting Chemicals can be read in full on the above website. Another informative article on bottled water by Dr. Mercola is "Bottled Water poisons your body one swallow at a time" Jan. 15th, 2011. Dr Mercola also writes a monthly newsletter which can be read online.

Chemicals In The Home

Everyday Household And Cleaning Products Are Implicated to birth defects

We have become desensitized to the products used in the home these days and need to know just what dangerous chemicals are lurking in these products that we are subconsciously inhaling. Cleaning and laundry products, caustic oven cleaning products, and highly perfumed air fresheners, etc. are widely used today and it maybe time people looked for safer chemical-free alternatives.

Fragrances Are Also Implicated In Birth Defects

Those eye-catching, highly perfumed fragrances used widely today may not be as innocent and harmless as they seem.

KLAUS FERLOW, HMHHA Author, research writer, founder of NEEM Research , writes:

FRAGRANCE – A GROWING HEALTH AND ENVIRONMENTAL HAZARD, *Klaus Ferlow*, HMH – 09/2007.

FRAGRANT CHEMICAL EXPOSURE IS HAZARDOUS TO EVERYONE

"Fragrances contain large amounts of phthalates, a group of toxic chemicals that are known oestrogen and testosterone hormone disruptors."

"A recent study suggests that diethyl phthalates, commonly used in fragrances and other personal care products damages the DNA of sperm which can lead to infertility, may be linked to miscarriages and birth defects and may lead to cancer and infertility in their offspring".

PHTHALATES have been associated with thyroid disorders, premature breasts developments in baby girls and abnormal sexual developments in male foetuses and infants (hypospadias and undescended testicles)."

"Especially vulnerable are foetuses, children, reproductive-age people and asthmatic, allergic and chemically-injured people (MCS – Multiple Chemical Sensitivity)

The remainder of this informative article can be read in full at the above website.

Perfumed Soaps And Candles Are Implicated In Birth Defects

Do you remember when bathroom soaps smelt like soaps? That was many years ago when fragrances had a delicately perfumed soapy aroma. It is hard to find the same type of decorative bathroom soaps today that are reasonably priced and with the old-fashioned soapy smell. Today the market is flooded with overpowering, headache inducing soaps and highly perfumed decorative candles enveloped in chemicals. You only have to walk pass stores selling soaps and candles and the overpowering odour escapes onto the footpaths. The odour is doubly overpowering when you enter the stores. So if stores sell highly perfumed soaps AND CANDLES, it is a double whammy for employees, meaning the employees working in these stores day after day are vulnerable and very exposed to these environmental toxins contained in soaps AND candles. I hate to think what the long term health effects are of store employees who work in those industries.

Highly-perfumed candles do not get off the hook either. A candle maker told me there are seven known carcinogens in perfumed candles. Exceptions to these are bees wax and soy candles.

In the HAZARDS OF SCENTS, Klaus Ferlow says:

"Most fragrant oils used to scent candles, soaps and myriad other products are very hazardous to your health. " Fragrance oils are combinations of synthetically manufactured chemicals designed to "mimic" the aroma of natural materials. Far from "natural" 95% of the chemicals found in these oils are synthetic compounds derived from petroleum, and include chemicals such as benzene derivatives, aldehydes, and others capable of causing cancer, birth defects, central nervous system disorders (CNS) and allergic reactions. Today, fragrances are marketed to an unsuspecting public who think that these scents are "natural". Even unscented and fragrance-free products can contain masking scents to "mask" the smell of other ingredients".

For eye-opening information, read enviroblog's 3, 163 ingredients hide behind the word "fragrance." Enviroblog is written by the Environmental working Group, an organization well worth supporting.

Alcohol Is Implicated In Birth Defects

The truth about the dangers of alcohol consumption by mothers (and FATHERS-to-BE) is now being discovered thanks to researchers and health experts.

TRUTH ABOUT DRINKING IN
PREGNANCY/News.com.au

This article is taken from the Body and soul on
15th December, 2013

Website
http://www.news.com.au/lifestyle/parenting/truth-about-drinking-in-pregnan...1/05/2014

"The advice from experts is clear: there are no "safe" level of alcohol consumption in pregnancy. But that message becomes impacted by a lot of human factors."

"More and more is being understood about foetal alcohol spectrum disorder (FASD), an umbrella term for a range of physical, developmental delay and is estimated to affect between 2 and 7 per cent of all births."

"This isn't a condition that's only found in disadvantaged pockets of the community, because drinking isn't confined to socio-economic groups, explains Elizabeth Elliott, a professor of paediatrics and child health at the University of Sydney."

"What we do know is that women who don't drink any alcohol during pregnancy face no risks of (this kind of) damage to their foetus," she says. Frequent, high intakes of alcohol and particularly binge drinking, increases the risk."

"What we don't know is the risk to an individual pregnancy. Each pregnancy is different and every woman's body responds differently to alcohol consumption because of a range of factors such as age, body composition, genetics and prior disease."

"So, she strongly advises that expecting and trying-to-conceive women apply the precautionary principle as recommended in Australia's national alcohol guidelines that "not drinking alcohol is the safest option".

"However, that's where some of these factors come in".

"Despite living in an age of highly accessible contraception, almost 50 per cent of pregnancies in Australia are unplanned. Add to that another contemporary issue of the sharp increase in young women binge drinking, and the message of having an alcohol-free pregnancy becomes blurred".

"A new study from Newcastle University has revealed that 8 out of 10 expectant mums drink alcohol during pregnancy – 64 percent higher than found in other Australian studies"

"This follows survey results released last year by the foundation for Alcohol Research & Education which found that 47 per cent of Australian women interviewed consumed alcohol while pregnant before knowing they'd conceived and almost 20% per cent drank alcohol after confirmation of their pregnancy."

More Revealing Information On The Dangers Of Alcohol Consumption Before And During Pregnancy

FATHERS-TO-BE WHO CONSUME ALCOHOL CANNOT ESCAPE RESPONSIBILITY

MALE DRINKING LINKED TO FETAL ALCOHOL SYNDROME

The article below is written by Nature World News on Feb. 17th, 2014

http://newsroom.taylorandfrancisgroup.com/news/press-release/fathers-drinking-also U7QI97GDGZ9-responsible-for-foetal-disorders#)

and

http://www.tandfonline.com/doi/full/10.1080/197683 54.2013.865675.#.U7QI bgDgz8)

"It is well established that maternal alcohol consumption is a risk factor of foetal alcohol syndrome (FAS). However, new research reveals that PATERNAL drinking may be a cause of FAS, as well."

"The study, published in Animal Cells and systems, researchers exposed one group of male mice to varying concentrations of alcohol and exposed one control group to saline. After being exposed to alcohol or saline the mice were mated and their offspring studied. The findings revealed that PATERNAL ALCOHOL CONSUMPTION can directly affect foetal development."

"In children, FAS causes significant problems such as retarded intellect, stunted growth and nervous system abnormalities, social problems and isolation, according to the press release announcing the findings".

"Of all the substances of abuse (including cocaine, heroin and marijuana), alcohol produces by far the most serious neuro-behavioural effects in the foetus," reads the Institute of Medicine's report to Congress in 1996. ...About 40,000 babies born with FAS each year, costing the nation up to $6 billion annually in institutional and medical costs."

"In the study, a number of foetuses fathered by MALES EXPOSED TO ALCOHOL suffered abnormal organ development or brain development. The foetuses fathered by the males exposed to saline had healthy development."

"These results have led the author to believe that alcohol consumption affects genes in sperm that are responsible for normal foetal development."

"Previously, fathers' drinking habits showed no repercussions in their unborn children. This research provides the first definitive evidence that preconception drinking habits by MEN can cause significant foetal abnormalities in their children".

"However, the mechanisms of paternal alcohol exposure causing certain transgenerational toxicities remain to be defined," concluded the study+

Over-Consumption Of Alcohol In Pregnancy – A Link To Downs Syndrome

There are still too many babies being born with Downs Syndrome, about 60-70 babies born in Australia each year while in the United States about 6,000 babies each year are being born with Downs Syndrome, according to the Centre for disease Control and Prevention (CDC) Even given the enormous size of the American population this number is quite staggering.

There has been some research as to what causes Downs Syndrome in newborn babies, some researchers think over consumption of alcohol by mothers AND fathers- to- be can be responsible for rising instances of Downs Syndrome. Another theory is that mothers-to-be have a folate deficiency (green vegetables) in their diet, (according to the Mayo clinic) or a diet lacking in green vegetables and healthy nutrients whilst pregnant; but there is no conclusive evidence of that fact; maybe it is a combination of many factors, faulty diet, light or heavy use of alcohol by both the mothers and fathers to-be and light or heavy smoking and then throw in light or heavy use of drugs like marijuana and methamphetamines, and cocaine, and then consequently there could be a lethal cocktail of birth defects disasters waiting to unfold at birth?

More investigative research needs to be carried out so BOTH parents-to-be know exactly where they stand with regard to drinking alcohol, and taking drugs and adopting a healthy diet and will hopefully act in a responsible manner, for the long-term health of their unborn child/children, before they contemplate the very important step of starting a family.

Illicit Drugs Are Implicated With Birth Defects In Newborn Babies As More And More Women Smoke Cannabis During Pregnancy

Many women (and men) smoke marijuana and other illicit drugs regularly and especially during pregnancy, for relaxation purposes and to escape stress in their lives, sometimes called "recreational drugs or party drugs" but their future life will be far from a party because of their reckless and dangerous behaviour nor do they not realise or understand the permanent physical damage their irresponsible and damaging habit can have on their unborn child/children.

Using Cannabis
Can Cause Birth Defects
In The Unborn Child

CANNABIS USE AND PREGNANCY

According to the National Cannabis and Information Centre (NCPIC).

Go to
http://ncpic.org.au/ncpic/publications/factsheet/articl
e/cannab. 4/10/2013

"Cannabis is the most commonly used illicit drug amongst women of reproductive age or by women who are pregnant.

"Even though there has been little research into the effects of cannabis use upon the unborn child, it is strongly recommended that pregnant women AND THEIR PARTNERS do not use alcohol or any other drug due to the potential harmful effects on the developing baby".

"Can cannabis use affect fertility?"

"Heavy use of cannabis has been linked to decreased fertility in both men and women. In females, there is evidence that cannabis use may disrupt the menstrual cycle. In males, cannabis is thought to decrease sperm quality and testosterone levels. It is also thought to decrease the ability of sperm to move quickly and has been linked to sperm abnormalities."

"These factors can make it difficult for a woman to become pregnant."

"Can cannabis use affect pregnancy?"

"THC (delta-9-teteahydrocannabinol), the main psychoactive ingredient in cannabis, is known to pass from the mother to the developing foetus through the placenta. This means that the foetus is affected by any amount of cannabis taken by the pregnant woman, placing it at a greater risk of complications occurring. The effect of the passive inhalation of cannabis as a result of breathing in the smoke of others is not clear, but it should be avoided."

"Any form of smoking can disrupt the supply of oxygen and nutrients to the foetus, which can result in restrictions to the growth of the foetus (including overall length, foot length, head size and body weight) and in rare cases, premature birth, miscarriage and stillbirth".

"Can cannabis use affect the baby?"

"There is some evidence that women who use cannabis during pregnancy are more likely to give birth to babies with lower birth weight, delayed commencement of breathing, an increase in features similar to those found in foetal alcohol syndrome, exaggerated startle response, tremors, poorer eyesight, poorer ability to adapt to new aspects of the environment, and a "hole in the heart" (ventricular septal defect)"

"Other studies have found that in the first six months of life, babies who have been exposed to cannabis in utero are also at a greater risk of developing asthma, chest infections, and other breathing problems such as wheezing."

"Research suggests that at ages three to four years, children of mothers who used cannabis while pregnant have poorer verbal, memory and reasoning ability; poorer motor skills and shorter length of play; and are more likely to be fearful, impulsive, inattentive, hyperactive and delinquent. These difficulties appear to persist to age 10 years, when they may be accompanied by increased depression and anxiety, along with reading and spelling problems and general underachievement at school. Such defects may also continue into adolescence and early adulthood, along with an increased risk of initiation to tobacco and cannabis use"

"In addition, there exists some evidence that mothers' cannabis use during pregnancy increases the risk of their children developing childhood cancers, including non-lymphoblastic leukaemia, rhabomyosarcoma (a rare, highly malignant tumour that can occur anywhere in the body), and astrocytoma (a type of brain tumour)."

"Preliminary research suggests that FATHERS' CANNABIS USE IN THE YEAR PRIOR TO THEIR CHILDRENS' BIRTH is associated with an increased risk of rhabdomyosarcoma in their children, and that FATHERS' cannabis use during conception, pregnancy or postnatally is associated with an increased risk of Sudden Infant Death Syndrome (SIDS) in their infants. Furthermore some research suggests that children of fathers who experience cannabis dependence at least at some point in their lifetimes are more likely to experience negative outcomes during childhood, such as poor attachment relationships with their caregivers and psychosocial impairments, including depression and conduct problems."

"Can cannabis use affect breast-milk?"

"When a breastfeeding mother uses cannabis, THC passes into the breast-milk and thus into the baby, where it can be stored in the baby's fatty tissue for several weeks."

"Using cannabis while breastfeeding may cause the baby to be unsettled and disrupt feeding cycles. As a result, cannabis use should be avoided when breastfeeding."

Can using cannabis impact on pregnancy care?

Other problems can be experienced by pregnant women using cannabis because they are less likely to disclose their use of cannabis to healthcare workers. "The stigma associated with their use, as well as fear, guilt and shame about what they may have exposed their unborn baby to, may prevent these women from giving a full history to their obstetricians or midwives.

This may impact on the quality of care for both the woman and her developing baby, as healthcare workers do not have a complete history".

What help is available?

"Women who are pregnant or who are planning to become pregnant as well as their partners, should be advised to stop using cannabis. Continued use should be discussed with a general practitioner, specialist or midwife who can provide help and support to cut down or quit cannabis use or refer patients on to specialist alcohol and other drug services."

Factsheet published August 1, 2008. Updated October 1, 2011.

Cocaine And Methamphetamines (Ice) Are Also Implicated

DRUG USE AND PREGNANCY
NEW LAWS WILL SEE BABIES TAKEN FROM
ADDICTED OR ABUSED MOTHERS
WHO REFUSE TO SEEK HELP

The article below is taken from the Sunday
Telegraph from Staff Writers on November16th, 2013

The link is
http://www.dailytelegraph.com.au/news/nsw/new-laws-will-se... 5/03/2014

"BABIES will be taken away at birth from drug-addicted or abused mothers who refuse to seek help, under new state laws that will kick in while the child is still in the womb."

"NSW Health does not record the number of babies born with drug addictions; however in the three years to 2011 John Hunter Hospital on the Central coast recorded 238 babies born with an addiction to substances including heroin, cannabis and amphetamines.

Jodie is a foster mother with Barnardos and has cared for 27 drug-addicted babies."

"DEFENCELESS TINY ADDICTS, NURTURED WITH LOVE: It is the sound of their cry, a piercing, distinctive scream that can only come from a baby withdrawing from drug-addiction."

"It's a different cry, it's a heartbreaking cry, you can't describe it but when you hear it you can tell it's not a normal baby cry," Jodie, 46, a Barnardos foster carer who has cared for 27 addict-babies, said."

"Their little knees are up into their stomach and they're screaming. You can walk the floor for six or seven hours with baby crying continuously – they're in pain."

"When she first started fostering newborns 12 years ago, babies with an addiction were almost non-existent."

"Today, they are routinely in her care. Her last seven babies were all withdrawing from drugs spanning from methamphetamines to heroin to cannabis."

"She picks them up from hospital, takes them home and immediately begins administering doses of morphine, which they need every four hours that can continue for up to four months."

"I've had cases where they've got infections in their toes, under their armpits from the withdrawals."

"They're not like your normal cuddly baby, they're very stiff and in a fair bit of pain."

"Jodie says the happy side to fostering is that children leave her and live happy and healthy lives." (Source: News Limited)

"Once they're off (their addiction), all of them (have) become like a normal child. It's very rewarding to see them at the end of it".

There is a new scourge recently receiving publicity affecting body-conscious young men (and women) who will do anything to achieve the perfect bodies they desire, either to have the upper edge in sporting prowess or males wanting to develop a perfectly buffed body to attract the opposite sex, will stop at nothing for a better than perfect body with abnormally bulging muscles, regardless of knowing or even caring about the frightening consequences ahead of them in the near future or in later life – ANABOLIC STEROIDS

Steroids Linked To Cancer, Self-Harm, Birth Defects

Sabra Lane
Updated Thurs.1st Nov. 2007

Go to
http://www.abc.net.au/news/2007-11-01/steroids-linked-to-ca... 8/03/2014

Professor Giselher Spitzer from Humbolt University in Germany has conducted much research and studies over the years and writes on Anabolic Steroids and its side-effects:

"During the 1970s and 1980s, the former East Germany conducted a state-sanctioned program administering anabolic steroids to its athletes."

"Now the horrific consequences of the doping program are beginning to emerge."

"A study of 52 of the athletes has revealed that not only do they have serious health issues, BUT THEIR CHILDREN HAVE HIGH RATES OF PHYSICAL AND MENTAL DEFORMITIES".

"And a quarter of the athletes suffer from cancer."

"The study was the first to analyse the long-term health consequences of East Germany's doping program on both athletes and their children."

"Initially 60 athletes were involved, but by the project's end, one had died and seven others withdrew from the study because of psychological problems."

"Associate Professor Giselher Spitzer from Humbolt University investigated the 52 remaining athletes and their 69 children."

"None of the athletes had known that they were taking anabolic steroids."

"Associated Prof. Spitzer says most of the children have disabilities.

"YOU HAVE 69 CHILDREN WHO SURVIVED THE BIRTH, AND MANY OF THEM ARE DAMAGED OR HAVE SOME DAMAGE, ESPECIALLY IF THE MOTHER WAS DRUGGED - IF THE FATHER WAS DRUGGED THERE ARE NOT SO MANY SIDE EFFECTS ON THE SECOND GENERATION," HE SAID.

"He says there was also a high cancer rate among the athletes themselves."

Associate Professor Spitzer says the lesson from the research is that doping is a danger to health.

"That's the first step. There is NO healthy doping," he said.

"Every doping agent, every doping pharmaceutical has side effects. We see that very clearly.

"The message is your children will be damaged by that practice."

"Many athletes, or many body builders for example, fitness athletes, say, 'It is my body, and I'll do what I want'."

"IT IS NOT THE TRUTH, IT'S NOT ONLY YOUR BODY, IT IS THE SECOND GENERATION, AND WE DON'T KNOW WHAT WILL BE OF THE THIRD GENERATION."

"Professor Giselher Spitzer hopes the research can be used to help athletes to avoid history repeating itself."

The complete article can be read in full on line at the beginning of the above article.

It has been documented that any steroid use can give people mood swings and can get very scaringly aggressive and sometimes violent. People in that category can be sportsmen, athletes and body builders and other people in general.

In conclusion to this section, there needs to be Health Educators and people working for Drug and Alcohol centres and Health Departments to go into schools, both primary and secondary, when children are most vulnerable, to speak to students warning about the dangers of using anabolic steroids, as children are getting into this dangerous practice younger and younger (some as young as eleven or twelve) especially young boys, need to be made aware, along with their parents, of the horrific consequences to their health, not only for the present but most importantly for the future when they plan to start a family, anabolic use which states above can cause serious birth defects in their offspring.

I have seen images of some rather scary male bodies who have overused steroids to the point where their muscles are abnormally super-huge and very exaggerated, bursting out of their shirts, looking scaringly aggressive.

More scary research has been well documented that steroid use while pregnant or before falling pregnant can cause the unborn child to be born with male secondary sex characteristics in a female and female sex characteristics in a male. Such people have been termed "intersex" or transgender.

Long Term Steroid Use Can Cause Specific Birth Defects

Long term steroid use can cause birth defects such as abnormal levels of sex hormones in the developing foetus of pregnant women who are taking steroids. These defects include mental retardation and pseudohermaphroditism, which means the baby, is born with both male and female sex features. Babies born with both male and female sexual organs may seem to have male genitals but have female reproductive organs in the pelvis or the reverse is obvious that a female baby may have the appearance of a female, but have one or maybe more testicles in the pelvis cavity. This condition is called Hypospadias in boys and girls. In relation to this there are instances where some males can be born with normal sized breasts at first but as they get older their breasts start developing into large breasts resembling a woman's shape and size. Some transgender males take the radical step to have breast reduction surgery to align with the feelings that they are a man trapped in a woman's body. Some males, (and females) after much consideration take the final step with sex transition surgery in an attempt to define their gender.

Could it be that steroid use before or during pregnancy can cause some babies to be born transgender or intersex, or other theories. There are some theories which suggest that mothers-to-be suffering with depression or other complaints during pregnancy were given synthetic hormones in the form of medication and these hormones containing oestrogen or testosterone might have caused hormone disruption and abnormalities in sexual organs at birth. More investigative research needs to be done.

More information can be found at Organisation Intersex International Australia at oii.org.au.

What Causes Homosexuality?

Soy Products Are One Factor Coming Under Scrutiny

There is much research conducted at the moment that mothers-to-be who consume soy products whilst pregnant could be placing the sexuality of their new-born infant at risk. Could this be one of the reasons for the rising instances of homosexuality? There was and still are Health Institutions who recommend we eat a lot of food products containing soy for good health. Most of this advice has turned out to be bad advice. Some researchers suggest excessive amounts of soy products can sometimes cause cancer?

One being, Jim Rutz, a preacher, Freelance Writer and Columnist for World Net Daily, (who sadly has now deceased) has done much research on the subject of consuming soy products interfering with sexuality, and possibly being one of the causes of Cancer, has written informative and comprehensive articles on the subject which is called: THE SHOCKING EFFECTS OF SOY ON BOTH SEXES, dated Dec.12th, 2006.

As there is limited room for all of the whole articles to be written in this chapter it can be read online in its entirety.

There are some schools of thought which think that there are other factors that could be responsible for a baby to be born homosexual, (the politically correct word now being "gay" or lesbian) such as genetic factors or environmental influences, such as a weak or absent father, a violent or alcoholic or drug addicted parent/parents, a dysfunctional family life or a lack of parental or family harmony. There are other reasons such as pregnant mothers-to-be taking medications for different ailments that can disrupt hormones causing sexual differences in their unborn children. Sometimes people can be born bi-sexual, that is having a sexual interest in males and or females, maybe because of a lack of suitable sexual partners of the same sex, or just experimenting, or some just like to be trendy and brag that they are bi-sexual, or genuinely interested in both sexes, or other unexplained reasons. More research needs to take place.

Solvents Are Implicated In Fertility And Transgender Tendencies

There is research done at The European Agency for Safety & Health (OSHA) states that the workplace where people are working in factories with high chemical pollution from solvents from the dry cleaning industry, cabinet makers and people making furniture, etc. can be responsible for birth defects in children and even transgenerational tendencies, but these traits are not visible straight away. (Go to OSHA Occupational risks at work – children's health to see the many occupations at risk.

John Archer, water expert and author, goes a little further in the 3rd chapter of his book, *The Water you*

Drink, how safe is it? where he writes about drinking tap water and the horrific sexual consequences on fish and animal life and humans alike.

Autism – A Once Rare Birth Abnormality, But Becoming A More And More Common Birth Defect

Autism or also known as Autism Spectrum Disorder is now an everyday occurrence in newborn-babies and develops in young children that was practically unheard of the 1940s, why is it so common now?

Below are several passages taken from an interview by Dr. Joseph Mercola with Dr Natasha Campbell-Mcbride:

"In this interview Dr. Campbell-Mcbride presents a truly fascinating and elegant description of the foundational conditions that contribute to Autism along with a pragmatic approach to help circumvent and stem the autism epidemic, the key is in the GUT.

"Dr Mcbride has a full time medical practice in the United Kingdom where she treats children and adults with autism, learning difficulties, neurological disorders, psychiatric disorders, immune disorders and digestive problems. Here she shares her insights about "Gut and Psychology Syndrome (GAPS) the same title of her book which she has written herself. She says that children with GAPS can be particularly prone to vaccine damage and the GAPS Nutritional programme; a natural treatment for Autism, ADHD, dyslexia, dysprasia, depression and schizophrenia."

"Dr. Natasha Campbell-McBride is a medical doctor with a post-graduate degree in Neurology. She worked as a neurologist and a neurosurgeon for several years before starting a family. When her OWN first child was diagnosed with autism at the age of three she was surprised that her own profession had no answers."

Back in 1984, when she graduated from medical school, autism was an exceptionally rare disorder with a prevalence of about 1 in 10,000. "By the time I graduated from Medical School I had never seen an autistic individual," she says. To be honest the first autistic child I encountered was my own. Five years ago we were diagnosing one child in 150, which is about a 40-fold increase in incidences. Now in Britain and in some countries we are diagnosing one child in 66. The rates are similar in the United States, Australia and New Zealand as well. She quietly delved into research looking for an answer for her son, and ended up getting a second postgraduate degree in human nutrition. As a result of her work her son fully recovered and is NO LONGER autistic"

I recommend reading of her book "Gut and Psychology Syndrome, (GAPS)" by Natasha Campbell-McBride.

Many doctors treating children diagnosed with Autism blame the often behavioural problems of the children on the parents and say that "bad parenting" is one of the causes and then prescribe medication to try to calm the child down. This is only a part of the problem and not the long term solution to autism and behavioural problems.

THERE ARE VARYING DEGREES OF AUTISM

Autism Spectrum Disorder comes in varying degrees ranging from mild forms of the disease to severe cases of autism where some children have totally uncontrollable and screaming behaviour, creating much stress and heartache for the parents of such children, because they are so difficult to control. Other symptoms are where children do not show any emotion when hugged or kissed, or cannot participate in normal childhood activities or sports.

Autism is now classed as a "disability".

Some children are oblivious of what is going on around them and some children consequently need to go to "special needs" schools. There are more severe cases of autism where children cannot speak at all, which causes a lot of heartache for their parents; these children need understanding and extra care, which can be very emotionally and financially draining for their parents. Many parents are at their wits' end trying to find answers to this quite common and heart-breaking syndrome in their children, even after many years of looking to find doctors who can give solutions to this perplexing disability? Unfortunately autistic traits can continue into adulthood, often undiagnosed, with people having anger management issues.

A TOXIC DIGESTIVE SYSTEM MAY BE THE CULPRIT

Diet and proper nutrition must not be overlooked and are needed to help solve the whole problem. Another theory by researchers of Autism is if an unsuspecting mother-to-be has a toxic digestive system, it can be passed down from the prospective mother onto the unborn child, causing serious digestion issues to that child and causing autistic tendencies. There are other health researchers who have discovered that mothers-to-be who have been prescribed Anti-depressants or other medications during their pregnancies have delivered babies with signs of Autism.

It is becoming more clearer to me with today's emphasis on take-away and processed foods, and less importance on healthy eating, mothers (and fathers-to-be) may need to spend more time and pay more attention to their diet and healthy food preparation, before contemplating starting a family.

I would like to add a story of a friend of mine who had a four year old girl who was usually very well behaved, but with occasional behavioural problems, and throwing tantrums. The mother, noticed when the child had eaten snack and junk foods and foods containing artificial colourings and flavourings like jellies, sweets, and snack foods, etc. this child would have bouts of screaming and throwing tantrums, similar traits to that of an autistic child, which were quite unbearable and generally unexplained behaviour, seeing that the child was usually quiet and well-behaved. The mother observed that the child was constipated that is she hadn't had a bowel motion in several days and noticed that the child also had a high fever, her behaviour which was usually that of a happy child, became unbearable, and disobedient, with accompanying tantrums. The fever always seemed to accompany the bad behaviour. Finally the mother realised the child's diet and her behaviour could be linked, so she firstly gave the child a mild laxative, cut out all the junk foods, and served more fruit and vegetables with meals of soups and green vegetables and drinking more fluids (filtered water preferably) and adding more fibre and fluids to her diet, and by cutting out the chemicals and artificial flavourings in her diet, her behaviour settled down and consequently had regular bowel movements again. From that point her hyperactive behaviour disappeared and the child became very calm and well behaved again. Sometimes there can be a fine line between Autism and ADHD Attention Deficit Hyperactive Disorder.

THERE IS A COMMON LINK WITH DIET TO AUTISM

Health Researchers have noticed there that children with autistic tendencies who refuse to eat green vegetables or healthy foods, only wanting to eat starchy carbohydrates, snack or junk or processed foods, pizzas, hamburgers, etc. sugary drinks included. This kind of diet only seems to fuel their autistic behaviour. One would think that the lack of green vegetables and healthy foods must affect the brains of special needs children in an adverse way, causing autistic tendencies. As well as autistic people not eating vegetables, it should be noted that less than 4% of Australians are eating enough vegetables and legumes, according to media reports. This statistic suggests that all parents should take a good hard look at their own diets by increasing their own fruit and vegetable intake. Children learn by good example. More research into the diets of autistic children needs to take place.

Parents also need to make sure their children are adequately hydrated by ensuring they are drinking a lot of filtered water, the same way they should be observing their own fluid intake. A lack of water may adversely affect childrens' behaviour? Fizzy or sugary fruit juices may also fuel their bad behaviour? By applying simple measures like the above and having an awareness of what children are eating, along with more fibre, parents can go a long way in alleviating or even curing their childrens' mild or severe Autism.

Food Intolerances Are Also Implicated With Unruly Behaviour In Children

Hyperactivity and ADHD are also very common behavioural problems with children in society today, sometimes continuing into adolescence if unchecked and can sometimes lead to crime, if not properly diagnosed and the diet not addressed accordingly, causing much angst for parents. All too often doctors are too quick to reach for their prescription pad prescribing medication which only sometimes just bandaids the problem and can have serious side effects.

According to Wikipedia, Dr. Ben Feingold a famous American doctor, a Paediatric Allergist, was one of, if not the first to discover hyperactivity and ADHD in children was caused by foods containing food colourings and flavours and artificial flavourings. Dr.. Feingold wrote one of several books in the 1970s, one titled "Why your child is hyperactive" and "The Feingold Cookbook"

Closer to home in Australia, Dr Robert Buist, another notable well known and respected Nutritional Biochemist also wrote several books in the 1980s titled "Food Intolerance" and "Food Chemical Sensitivity" and "The Cholesterol Myth". Dr. Buist has a degree in BIOCHEMISTRY and a PHD in Medicinal Chemistry from Macquarie University as well as degrees in chiropractic and naturopathic medicine and has done numerous TV interviews and is a dynamic speaker, a testimony I can attest to myself, having heard him deliver talks on many occasions, at various venues. Dr. Buist lectures extensively both in Australia and overseas – among his many achievements.

Caffeine Is Also
A Culprit In Pregnancy

COFFEE IS IMPLICATED IN PREGNANCY
By *Dr Joseph Mercola*

Mercola, H.C. Retrieved Jan. 3, 2009
Dr. Mercola's comments:
http://articles.mercola.com/sites/articles/archives/200
9/01/03

Another article by Dr. Joseph Mercola on the risks of women drinking whilst pregnant states:

"HOW CAFFEINE DURING PREGNANCY CAN DAMAGE YOUR BABY"

"I've been warning of the dangers of caffeine to pregnant women for years.

"Amidst the ever changing often conflicting information about what constitutes a "safe" amount of caffeine for expectant mothers, it has always been my position that NO amount of caffeine during pregnancy is safe. As this study points out – and this is a significant finding for mainstream research – the equivalent of just TWO cups of coffee during pregnancy may affect your child's heart function, and if your baby is male, could also lead to a weight problem."

"Take note that's the equivalent of two cups of coffee during the entire pregnancy – not two cups of coffee per day".

How Caffeine Affects Your Unborn Baby

"Caffeine is an addictive, stimulant drug that passes easily through the placenta to the developing foetus. It is also transferred through breast milk."

"In babies (Newborn and unborn) the half-line of caffeine is extended. It stays in your baby longer, and a developing foetus has no ability to detoxify caffeine."

"Research has shown that ingesting caffeine during pregnancy can result in a wide range of problems for you and your baby including:

- Increased risk of miscarriage
- Low birth weight
- Birth defects such as clef palate
- Increased risk of Sudden Infant Death syndrome (SIDS)
- Decreased levels of iron and calcium in the expectant mother"

Coffee And Pesticides

"Another good reason to eliminate caffeine while pregnant is the fact that coffee crops grown outside the US are heavily sprayed with pesticides."

"Pesticides have been linked to a host of health problems, including miscarriages and stillbirths".

Caffeine Sources

Coffee (even decaf coffee contains a few milligrams of caffeine)

- Tea
- Cola Drinks
- Energy Drinks
- Cocoa and chocolate
- Over the counter and prescription drugs (especially pain medications)

There are people who will say "well I drank a lot of coffee in my pregnancy many years ago and my children well all born healthy" BUT coffee is being drunk a lot stronger these days, which means more caffeine is being ingested like (short blacks and macchiatos) by more and more people, many younger than years previously, and more people have coffee machines at home, than in previous years, so coffee is being drunk more often at home and brewed much stronger. Coffee Shops are doing a roaring trade these days with people being seen everywhere, carrying take away cups of coffee with them (almost like a fashion accessory).

THERE IS RELATIVELY NEW EVIDENCE EMERGING ABOUT THE DANGERS OF THE INCREASING USE OF ELECTROMAGNETIC RADIATION BEING HARMFUL TO THE BODY IN TODAYS WORLD WITH PEOPLE USING MORE AND MORE DEVICES THAT EMIT RADIATION AND ALSO CHILDREN BEING INTRODUCED TO THEM YOUNGER AND YOUNGER.

OVEREXPOSURE TO RADIATION IS BEING IMPLICATED IN CANCER AND BIRTH DEFECTS IN BABIES AND YOUNG CHILDREN.

Reproduced from "The Force: living safely in a world of electromagnetic pollution" by Lyn McLean, published by Scribe Publications, 2011. Lyn McLean is also director of EMR Australia. Below are just a few passages from the above book:

Cell Phones And Male Fertility

"Use of cell phones decreases semen quality in men."
Dr. Ashok Agarwal

Lyn McLean writes "For decades, it has been known that electromagnetic radiation has the potential to interfere with fertility. During world war 11, sailors were known to willingly expose themselves to their ships' radar in order to enjoy its contraceptive advantages during shore leave."

"But now there's a new way in which men are irradiating themselves – by carrying a mobile phone in their trouser pockets. While the phone is turned on it is emitting microwaves, and that radiation is being absorbed by the sensitive reproductive organs located close by."

"There are literally dozens of studies that have found that mobile phone radiation can reduce sperm count and affect sperm quality. Most of these have found that it affects several aspects of sperm viability, including its motility (movement), morphology (shape and size) and vitality (potency). If any of these qualities are compromised, the sperm is less likely to successfully negotiate its way to the egg and achieve fertilisation."

"This could have serious implications for reproduction. Researchers in this field say that it may be 'potentially affecting both their fertility and the health and wellbeing of their offspring' that 'keeping the cell phone in a trouser pocket in talk mode may negatively affect spermatozoa and impair male fertility'; that 'RF-EMR from mobile phones negatively affect semen quality and may impair male fertility'.

"Dr. John Aitken is Laureate Professor in Biological Sciences at Australia's University of Newcastle and the Director of the Centre for Reproductive Science. He has published a number of studies during the past decade in which he has shown that mobile phone radiation reduced the viability of sperm. In 2009, he produced a ground breaking study that showed, for the first time, just how this effect could occur. Professor Aitken and his team exposed sperm to a mobile phone signal 1.8 GHz (the typical frequency a 3G mobile phone signal), and found that the sperm had reduced motility and vitality. In fact, mobile phone radiation caused the sperm's mitochondria to leak electrons, which resulted in oxidation. Oxidation is associated with DNA damage and infertility. The more radiation absorbed by the sperm, the greater the effects. On the basis of their results, Aitken's team recommended that 'men of reproductive age who engage in high levels of mobile phone use do not keep their phones in receiving mode below waist level'

"Are these phones becoming the contraceptive of the modern time – the radar of the twenty-first century? In case they are, men may well be advised to keep their mobile phones out of their trouser pockets".

"Other forms of microwave exposure have also been found to affect fertility. Doctor Weyandt from Pennsylvania State University found that artillerymen in the US army whose work was likely to expose them to microwaves had lower sperm counts and ejaculated lower levels of sperm than unexposed men. Several studies have also found testicular changes in mice exposed to EMR from microwaves."

Hands-Free Devices
Now Available

There are now safer options available when using a mobile or cell phone such as hands-free devices like head sets and phone mode options so phones do not come in direct contact with the head.

Cordless Phones
Are Also Implicated

McLean advises that cordless land line phones generate similar radiation exposure to that of mobile phones. She advises to limit radiation exposure with short phone calls or use a corded phone. I mostly use the speaker option on my cordless land line phones at home, especially when engaging in long conversations, and always keep the ear-piece a few inches away from my ear.

McLean also advises to keep cordless land line phones and mobile phones and computers out of bedrooms, of adults and children alike, as there can be much radiation present also disrupting much needed sleep.

Over Exposure To Computer Use In Pregnancy Is Implicated

"Because of possible association of EMFs with birth defects and miscarriage, consideration should be given to providing workers who are contemplating pregnancy in their families with the option of moving to duties other than screen-based work."

"Children may be more sensitive to EMFs than adults, so more stringent measurements and precautions should be taken if there is childcare in the workplace. School computer rooms, which may use old equipment in crowded conditions, should also receive rigorous attention".

Brain Tumors

Concerns About Radiation In Children

'The danger of brain tumours from cellphone use is highest in children and the younger a child is when he/she starts using a cellphone the higher the risk'

Lloyd Morgan

"Children are more vulnerable to the radiation from mobile phones for a number of reasons. They have thinner skulls, and therefore radiation is able to penetrate further into their heads. As children and foetuses grow, their cells are often dividing, and during this process they are more vulnerable to radiation. Because a child's head can be similar in size to the wavelength of mobile phone radiation, the radiation can resonate in their heads, causing a greater impact. Some mobile phones emit signals that lie in the range of alpha and delta brainwaves, the very brain patterns that are constantly changing in children up to the age of about 12, when the alpha rhythm becomes established."

BABIES AND YOUNG CHILDREN AT RISK

Mobile phone devices with inbuilt cameras seem to be very popular at the moment, being used to photograph babies and young children. New parents and other family members understandably want to photograph every single happening and progress of their precious offspring. I am rather concerned at this new current practice – can the radiation from these phones be absorbed into their little heads and bodies causing brain or other damage?? Research needs to be done.

McLean continues:
"While brain tumours have been the focus of many researchers, they are, of course, not the only problem that has been linked to mobile phone use. Mobile phone radiation has also been associated with low immunity, behavioural problems, and reduced fertility, among other health concerns."

"Even foetuses can be affected by the radiation from mobile phones. A joint study from Denmark and the United States surveyed the mothers of over 13,000 children who were aged seven between 2005 and 2006 and found that mothers who had used a mobile phone while they were pregnant were 54% more likely to have children with behavioural problems, such as hyperactivity and difficulties interacting with other children. In 2008, an Egyptian study found that pregnant women's use of mobile phones affected their unborn babies; the researchers measured increases in heart rate and decreased cardiac output in foetuses that had been exposed to mobile phones"

"For would-be fathers there is a further caution. A number of studies have now shown that men who use mobile phones have reduced sperm quality and mobility and an increased risk of fertility. It's worth keeping in mind that your sensitive reproductive organs may be absorbing the radiation if you carry a mobile phone in your hip pocket while it is turned on."

Microwave Ovens Radiation

There has been no definitive evidence that any or much exposure to microwave ovens is implicated in birth defects with microwave use but it is wise to err on the side of caution, even for good health in general, and try to restrict the use of the above, using a regular convection oven and hot plates, cooktops, or stoves as much as possible and only using a microwave oven as a back-up and only when it is unavoidable, whether pregnant or not.

McLean covers all areas of EMFs extensively in her book, The Force, including dangers from living near over-head power lines, Base Stations and Broadcast Towers, and the dangers of Wi-Fi computer use, iPads, and much more.

The above passages are just several paragraphs taken from Lyn McLean's book, "The Force". It is a very well written and informative book which raises awareness of new-age electromagnetic radiation and a book everyone needs to read, for their own health and the health of their children and loved ones.

Chapter 14

Water - What Are We Drinking?

There is much debate among the Medical Profession as well as the general public as to whether to drink tap water or filtered water or bottled water. I know one thing – I would not have had the success in my rapid cure of cancer if I had drunk tap water. Home-filtered water (Reverse Osmosis) is the best method of drinking water as it removes all heavy metals, chlorine, lead, fluoride, pesticides, herbicides, etc. Bottled water is popular, but a home-filtering system pays for itself in six months, when you consider what you spend on bottled water and having to lug it home on a regular basis. Once you have tasted drinking water from a Reverse Osmosis Home filtering System, it is hard to drink anything else; nothing comes close to the taste, even bottled water.

John Archer, Researcher, Author, and consumer Advocate, with a passionate interest in water issues, has written 22 books, several of them on water, so I will let an expert (John Archer) (rather than myself) explain the passages below, how important it is to know exactly what's in our drinking water. Below are many, informative, extensive writings taken from one of his books "The Water you drink, How Safe is it?"

Archer writes :

"Water authorities and health officials regularly assure us that our water is perfectly safe… but the truth is they don't really know if it is safe or not. In fact no one knows what "safe" means.

"If you ask water authority staff what they mean, they'll tell you that the water is measured against strict guidelines for water quality set by the National Health and Medical Research Council (NHMRC)."

Catchment Contaminants

"Crystosporidium is just one of the super bugs that infest our water catchments. Apart from sewage, there are many other serious sources of viral, parasite, and artificial oestrogen contamination. These include waste water from chicken processing plants, abattoirs, diaries and hospitals."

"From the Philippines comes a documented report of some of the horrendous side effects which can occur after drinking hormone-contaminated water. Little girls who drank from a creek downstream from a factory which killed and washed hormone-injected chickens were found to be growing breasts and beginning periods at the age of five".

"Even here in Australia and other western countries there is an increase in young girls developing breasts and menstruating younger and younger."

"Abattoir waste contains a ghastly mixture of parasites viruses associated with animal excrement, blood and intestines– the most insidious of these parasites, Crystosporidium – has already been found in Sydney and Melbourne drinking water and that of many rural areas (see Chapter 4). Medical wastes and waste water from hospitals contains a cocktail of natural and synthetic steroids found in oral contraceptives, anti-cancer drugs and other medications."

"Some or all of these activities are happening in our major water catchments, and as a result millions of invisible organisms and chemical compounds are passing unmonitored and undetected into our drinking water."

"In April 1993, 400,000 residents of Milwaukee, Wisconsin, fell ill with waterborne cryptosporidiosis, a gastroenteric disorder caused by a chlorine resistant parasite which passed undetected through the city's modern water treatment plant"

"In the same year research in Canada demonstrated that tap water which met all of the required health parameters would still cause a great deal of illness. In this trial, people who used reverse osmosis purifiers experienced 30% fewer gastrointestinal disorders than those who drank ordinary treated tap water."

"Is it merely a coincidence that 30% of the Lucky Country suffers from what's known as irritable bowel syndrome or IBS?

According to Dr. Stephen Juan: "It is estimated that about one-third of Australians suffer from this abdominal complaint. About 50 per cent of outpatients at hospital gastroenterology departments or clinics are there to seek treatment for IBS."

"The cause of this epidemic has not been established, but water-borne viruses and parasites are high on the list of possibilities."

Longevity And Vilacabambans

As mentioned in an earlier chapter about the longevity of the Vilacabambans, their longevity is again mentioned by John Archer in chapter 2, "The Fountain of Regeneration":

"Vilacabamba is a source of fascination to researchers investigating the phenomenon of longevity. In a village with a population of 814, 15 per cent are over 80 years old, 12 people exceed 100 years, and Jose Maria Roa is the oldest person in the Western Hemisphere. To put this in some sort of perspective, in the US only one person in every 1.7 million lives to 100 years or more. In Vilacabamba it's 1 in 68."

"Dr. Morton Walker who has made a detailed study of the area, concluded that the secret lay in minerals contained in the water from the spring which provides the village with drinking water. While each of the seven minerals has a specific life-giving and youth-enhancing function, our investigations kept coming back to the amazing fact that Vilacabambans are free of the diseases that usually cut short the lifespans of Westerners."

"Heart disease, for instance, is uncommon (and perhaps unknown in Vilacabamba). This, we believe, is due to the overall synergetic workings of the minerals in their drinking water."

"Ecuador is a long way away but healthy water which will enhance your well-bring may be closer at hand. Rainwater, mineral water, bottled water or home purified water are four options which will be discussed in the chapters which follow".

"For the moment, let's concentrate on the relationship between our health and the water we drink".

"The normal healthy body attempts to maintain a constant water level by a number of mechanisms. The one we're most familiar with is the sensation of thirst. In order to satisfy this need we go to the tap, but if the water tastes or smells even slightly offensive, we tend to put off drinking it and opt for something more palatable."

"Worse still we may become conditioned to ignore this early warning signal of physical distress."

"However, thirst is not always a good indicator of the body's need for water. In order to maintain proper hydration, adults require at least one and a half to two litres of water every day, about six to eight big glasses. That sounds simple enough to achieve, but because of the deteriorating quality of our tap water, involuntary dehydration has become a widespread condition, one which may have serious long-term medical consequences."

Many people find it difficult to drink the above amounts of water, but because tap water is so unpalatable, they make a rather unhealthy decision to instead drink other forms of fluids such as soft drinks or diet drinks or packaged fruit juices, not realising how much sugar or artificial sweeteners they are ingesting daily. Coffee is another unhealthy option where many people down several to many cups per day.

"According to the water expert Dr. Batmanghelidj, an age-dependent loss of the thirst sensation in humans can lead to dyspeptic pain, rheumatoid joint pain, angina pain, hypertension, asthma, allergy, raised cholesterol, chronic fatigue syndrome, and diabetes in the elderly."

"Dr. Batmanghelidj believes that many of these disorders can be exacerbated or even caused by dehydration. At first this may seem like an outrageous claim. In order to consider this, it's necessary to briefly outline the physical functions which water serves."

Are You Drinking Enough?

"There are three simple clinical signs." Dark yellow urine. Our kidneys are equipped with millions of filtering units that remove impurities and return the purified fluid to the bloodstream. Since filtration is the organ's first priority, it will continue its job even if this means producing very highly concentrated urine. Over a long period of time, dehydration can lead to the development of kidney stones, urinary tract infections, and other problems."

"Constipation. This bowel dysfunction is often one of the first signs that your water intake is inadequate. Because the rest of the body has a higher priority for water, the intestinal tract can be short-changed, and the result is hard stools. Unfortunately, few people heed this warning. Instead they usually rely on medication or patent remedies which force the rest of the body to return water from its own limited supply to the intestinal tract."

'Dry mouth' caused by decreased salivary gland function, can also result from low water intake. On the other hand, a person who drinks enough water seems not to need much during meals, since his or her saliva glands operate properly.

Treating Migraines

"In my personal experience, migraine headaches seem to be brought about by dehydration; excess bed covers that will not permit the body to regulate its temperature during sleep; alcoholic beverages initiating a process of cellular dehydration, particularly in the brain; dietary or allergy triggers for histamine release; excess environmental heat without water intake. Basically, migraines seem to be an indicator of critical body temperature regulation at times of 'heat stress.' Dehydration plays a major role in the precipitation of migraine headaches."

"The most prudent way of dealing with migraine is its prevention by the regular intake of water. Once migraine breaks the barriers, a cascade of chemical reactions will stop the body from further activity. At this time, one may be forced to take analgesic medications with copious water. Sufficient cold or iced water may of itself be able to cool the body (also the brain) from inside and promote closing of the vascular system everywhere. The excess dilation of the peripheral vessels might be the basic cause of migraine headache."

Water And Stress

"Depression and social stresses such as fear, anxiety and insecurity often lead us to indulge in alcohol, tranquillisers, coffee, cigarettes and other drugs in order to leave our distress behind. Under these circumstances we often forget our water intake. It has been suggested that depression and stress can themselves be the product of dehydration, as well as exacerbating it. Don't forget that your brain is 85% water and if deprived of even a small amount of its fluid requirements, thought processes and emotional stability are the first to be affected."

"Although alcohol, coffee, milk and flavoured drinks contain water, they do not adequately supply the body's needs. Do not count them as part of your daily water intake or you'll be short changing yourself. On the other hand, if you increase your water intake, you will probably decrease your consumption of other less vital fluids."

Time For A Drink

"If six to eight glasses of water is the minimum daily intake, the next question is when should you drink it? According to the experts, its best to replace fluid as your body eliminates it. In other words, there's no point in getting up in the morning and downing eight glasses all at once. Your kidneys would soon eliminate the excess, and it wouldn't be available when needed later in the day. However, after a night's sleep, your body is somewhat dehydrated, so you should start replacing water by drinking about two glasses at least fifteen minutes before you have breakfast. Once you've had your morning meal, wait a couple of hours to make sure the food has left your stomach, and then have another two glasses. Drink two or three more throughout the afternoon, and have one or two after supper. This adds up to a total of seven or more glasses of water during the course of your day."

"Two things are likely to happen if you follow this regimen. First your thirst will be quenched. Second, not only will you replace the fluids your body needs, but you'll do so with a liquid which is more health promoting than fluids like coffee or alcohol."

"The more I become acquainted with the mysteries of water, the more convinced I am that the water we drink is a significant factor in maintaining our personal and domestic harmony, as well as our health. We are, after all, the water we drink."

In the words of the poet Robert Frost: "Here are your waters and your watering place, Drink and be whole again beyond confusion."

"There are more than a thousand toxic pollutants which threaten the security of your water supply – water authorities test for thirty at most before assuring you that the water's safe."

"Think about that for a minute: hundreds of toxic chemicals, pesticides and weedkillers, viruses and parasites, some unknown, not even tested for, or even monitored."

Archer continues:

Safe Poison

"Let me introduce you to atrazine, the world's most widely used weedkiller. I first learned about atrazine from a woman who specialises in pesticides and their impacts, the ecologist, Dr. Kate Short. Kate's book Quick Poison, slow Poison: Pesticide risk in the Lucky Country, is a mine of information on the subject. She also produces an informative quarterly newsletter called Sentinel and the September 1995 issue was devoted to pesticides in drinking water; atrazine comes up for special mention".

"Atrazine is an organochlorine herbicide extensively used for agriculture and forestry. It's also commonly used in urban areas where it is sprayed all over the place – around railway reserves, roads footpaths, and domestic gardens, all the places where children play. It would be nice to know that it was safe, wouldn't it?"

"While your water authority considers atrazine a low-risk herbicide, 'safe' within their flexible definition, current research tells a different story. We are really gambling that atrazine will not affect our children as badly as it affects laboratory mice."

Kate Short's research indicates that: 'exposure to atrazine is associated with prostate, ovarian and breast cancer and also damages the endocrine system by functioning as a synthetic hormone disruptor. As a "hormone mimic" it can block, antagonise, compete with, or mimic hormones at a cellular level. This may lead to reproductive and endocrinal effects. Atrazine has also demonstrated cardiac toxicity in experimental animals. Exposure may lead to abdominal pain, impaired adrenal function, anaemia, dermatitis, diarrhoea, skin, eye and mucous-membrane irritation, nausea and vomiting. Long term impacts include weight loss, possibly anorexia, cardiac dilation, cancer; CNS excitation/depression, growth, retardation, prenatal damage, kidney damage, spleen haemorrhage, tremor. Long term exposure may also lead to rash or sensitisation.'

"How can you protect yourself? Atrazine in water is more difficult to get rid of than cancer, because it's a systemic poison. This means that its residues penetrate the flesh of fruit and vegetables. These residues cannot be washed off."

"Inside the plant tissue, the atrazine degrades and converts into what's called a metabolite, which is believed to pose the same threat to human health as does atrazine. Its toxicity levels are not known."

"The Europeans are cautious about pesticides like atrazine, because they seem to be doing something strange to the fish population.'

Something Fishy Going On

"W.C fields, alcoholically challenged comedian of the silent era, once said that he wouldn't drink tap water "because fish f....k in it'".

"That was back in the good old days. Now lots of fish in our rivers and seas appear to have lost interest in copulation. Some of them have developed interesting genetic mutations. Hermaphrodite fish have often been caught in Victoria's Port Phillip Bay, and a major British study has revealed that male fish downstream from sewage treatment plants are changing sex as a result of 'estrogenic chemicals which are not removed from the treated effluent".

"These chemicals, which mimic the effects of the female hormone, oestrogen, have recently been linked to a disturbing explosion of sexual abnormalities and disorders in animals and humans. These manifestations include panthers with undescended testes, alligators with abnormally small penises, bisexual seagulls, hermaphrodite fish, laboratory rats with scrambled reproductive systems. The effects of these rogue hormones are thought to include as well as any of the above, a lowering of the sperm count and consequent difficulty with conception, a doubling of testicular and prostate cancer in men and an increase in breast cancer in women."

"In some rural communities where high pesticide use has left residuals in drinking water, there have been reports of boys with abnormally small penises along with feminisation of males and masculination of females. Research into the reasons for this is continuing; Scientific American (October 1995) list atrazine and endosulfan as proven synthetic oestrogens."

"Both chlorine and organochlorines can produce synthetic oestrogens, and some scientists are as present investigating the effects on humans of chlorine compounds widely used in American and Australian agriculture, industry, and water treatment."

When nutrient-loaded water is exposed to heat, sunlight, and sluggish flow due to drought or too much irrigation extraction, significant changes may take place.

The Greening Of Our Water

"It was this explosive combination of factors which was responsible for the spectacular display of blue-green algae which appeared in the Darling River in November 1991. This was the largest algal bloom ever recorded in any river in the world. More than a thousand kilometres were affected, resulting in a State of emergency being declared in NSW for three weeks."

"Smaller outbreaks continue to occur throughout Australia with alarming frequency; Alarming because blue-green algae is a serious public health hazard."

Toxic Treatments

"For decades it has been assumed that small amounts of chlorine in drinking water are safe, but convincing evidence, largely unreported to the public, has been accumulating for years that shows correlations between chlorinated water and the onset of serious disease."

COLIN INGRAM,
THE DRINKING WATER BOOK, 1991
THE WATER OF FORGETFULNESS

"A couple of weeks ago a fellow water researcher sent me a card for my noticeboard. Two hardened-looking characters are sitting in a saloon bar – the dialogue goes like this:

Why do you drink?

To forget.

To forget what?

Err, I don't remember!

Hey, it worked!

Great! Let's have a drink to celebrate!

"Memory loss is on the increase in Australia and it's not just the aged and infirm who are at risk. Memory loss seems to be quite widespread amongst politicians, police commissioners, and failed entrepreneurs of the 1980s."

"Could it be the aluminium in their drinking water, I wondered?

"Many eminent medical men are now sure that aluminium is a key factor in the spread of Alzheimer's disease. There are about 120,000 Australians with advanced dementia, a figure that's due to double in fifteen years if we don't do something about it."

"Well, for once Sydney water is doing the right thing by its customers – at last it's going to stop putting aluminium in the drinking water."

"Why did Sydney decide to stop, you might ask? The answer is contained in a front page story in the Sydney Morning Herald of 30 March 1995."

'Memory Loss May Start with a Glass of Water' warned the headlines, as science and environment editor Bob Beale presented the following story.

"Sydney medical researchers have discovered what they say is the strongest link so far between Alzheimer's disease and the world's most widely used water-filtering chemical, alum."

"A team led by Dr. Judie Walton, of the Australian Institute for Biomedical Research, has shown that traces of dissolved aluminium in alum-treated drinking water may enter the brain – from as little as a single glass of water."

"Alum is the common name for aluminium sulphate, which is dissolved and used to find fine sediments for removal."

"Dr. Walton said yesterday that aluminium was a known neurotoxin , or nerve poison, and dissolved aluminium was the most toxic and 'bio-available' form of metal and therefore the most potentially damaging to humans."

"Dr. Walton, president of the International federation of Cell Biology, says there is more evidence that aluminium is involved in Alzheimer's disease than any other single factor."

"She called for a global review of the use of alum, saying the research suggested that the World Health Organisation's standards or maximum aluminium concentrations in drinking water – which apply in Australia – were probably 100 times too high."

John Archer's last words on the above topic of Alzheimer's disease are:

"And then for God's sake get yourself a good water purifier while you still remember what they look like."

Tap Water And Miscarriage

"It appears that there are other less obvious hazards as well. Two important studies have recently highlighted health problems associated with drinking treated tap water. Both are well known to the water industry, but have not been discussed with the general public."

"The first study deals with the connection between tap water and miscarriage, a link established in research carried out by the Californian Department of Health Services in Berkeley, California."

"In 1981 a routine collection of data on the State's drinking water and its effects on health led to the unexpected discovery that women throughout California who drank tap water had rates of miscarriage or spontaneous abortion three to four times higher than women who drank only bottled water."

"In 1988 the New York times published the following article called 'Puzzling findings on Bottled Water in Pregnancy'

"Californian health officials are planning further studies in an attempt to explain puzzling results that seem to suggest that tap water might contribute to miscarriages and birth defects."

"The Californian Department of Health Services reported last week that pregnant women who said they drank bottled water had fewer miscarriages than one would expect from birth statistics. These women also seem to have children with slightly fewer than the expected number of birth defects. Pregnant women who drank tap water had the expected number of miscarriages and children born with birth defects."

"Moreover, it was found that it did not matter what part of California a woman lived in. And despite local differences in the sorts of chemicals added to various drinking water supplies, no significant differences in miscarriage rated occurred. All tap waters seemed to show the mysterious miscarriage-producing effect."

"Four years later Dr. Shanna Swan and her colleagues from the California Health Department published the final results of their ten year research in

Epidemiology, March 1992. One startling study showed that 'no spontaneous abortions were identified among women who reported abstaining from tap water during pregnancy."

"The following month the Swan report was summarised in the Sydney Morning Herald by Stephen Juan, who made some additional observations:

"In addition, some data suggested that the more tap water a pregnant woman drank, the greater was her risk of miscarriage. As Dr. Swan and colleagues said 'Two glasses of tap water per day appeared to be riskier than one glass.'

Gastrointestinal Illness

"We've looked at the relationship between tap water and sexual abnormalities, and miscarriage, but can tap water also cause disease in our daily lives as well?

'Definitely, says Canadian water researcher Pierre Payment. Payment and two other researchers, Eduardo Franco and Jack Siemiatycki, set out to demonstrate that the conventional methods used to evaluate drinking water quality in Canada (and Australia) do not provide adequate assurances of safety."

"The study commissioned by the University of Quebec was conducted on 600 families. Half of those surveyed drank water which had been treated by the City of Montreal's modern treatment plant while the balance consumed the same water after further home treatment with a reverse osmosis purifier."

"The draft 1993 Australian Drinking water guidelines instructed water authorities that if Cryptosporidium is 'detected in a distribution system, then urgent steps (such as issuing 'boil water' notices) should be taken to prevent infections in the community, and detailed advice should be sought from health authorities'.

"If the Sydney event was an example of how health departments and water boards handle their responsibilities, it shows that there is much left to be desired."

"In my opinion, both the Water board and the Health Department deliberately deceived consumers and the media about the nature of a potential threat to public health."

"Cryptosporidium is considered by the US Environmental Protection Agency to be one of the three most common disease-causing organisms in the world and to be responsible for 25-30 per cent of diarrhoeal outbreaks where there is no other known cause."

"Cryptosporidium was found both in the Sydney catchment and the pipeline system; it did not magically disappear. Since there is no treatment barrier in place at present, there is no reason to believe that consumers are protected from the threat of a serious disease outbreak similar to that which occurred in Milwaukee."

The Great Fluoride Debate

Archer continues on the fluoride debate:

"The debate about the addition of fluoride to drinking water is an ongoing one and many books have been written in an effort to explain it. Space does not permit such long and reasoned arguments here, so I'll simply sum up the more obvious points made by others, starting with Dr. Charles Heyd, past president of the American Medical Association who wrote:

'The plain fact that fluorine is an insidious poison, harmful, toxic and cumulative in its effects, even when ingested in minimal amounts, which remain unchanged no matter how many times it will be repeated in print that fluoridation of (the) water is 'safe'.

"It appears that fluoridated water may be particularly unsafe for pregnant mothers because of its potential to damage the cells of the developing foetus."

"In a shocking report titled Increased Death rate in Chile Associated with Artificial Fluoridation of Drinking Water with Implications for Other countries, Professor Albert Schatz examined the incidence of congenital malformations, that is, malformations caused by faulty development, infection, or injury in the uterus."

"Professor Schatz presented figures which showed that 244 per cent more deaths resulted from congenital malformations in the city of Curico (fluoridated in 1953) from 1953 to 1963, than in the unfluoridated control town (which served as a comparison, where one factor is different, to test the results of an experiment) of San Fernando. Deaths from diseases of the digestive system were 50 per cent higher in fluoridated Curico and infant mortality rates were 69 per cent higher."

"In 1977, a year after this report was published, water fluoridation ceased in Chile."

"Most developed countries have either abandoned or rejected fluoridation because of many similar studies linking fluoride with cancer, genetic mutations, and long-term effects on enzyme production and the immune system."

"This leaves Australians with the most exposed population of any country in the world – more than 70 per cent of us drink fluoridated water. Brisbane is the only capital city without fluoridation."

Fluoride Fiasco
At Brisbane North Pine
Water Treatment Plant

Fluoride is toxic to most bodily systems. An incident on North Pine Water Treatment Plant in Brisbane in 2009 occurred when an overdose of fluoride tablets was added to the drinking water levels, which resulted in the death of a 2 yr. old boy. This lack of care was caused by the Water Authority's failure to adequately monitor fluoride water levels and then by not informing a previous Queensland Government in time, about the higher than normal doses of fluoride in the Water Supply.

Potential For Overdose

Attention Deficit Disorder Findings

LEAD ASTRAY

Archer continues on Lead in drinking water:

"Australian doctors say that they are at a loss to explain the ever-increasing rate of hyperactivity and learning difficulties now categorised as attention deficit disorder (ADD). The problem has been documented in many countries during the last 50 years."

"Children who are diagnosed as 'suffering' from ADD are usually prescribed stimulant medications like Ritalin or dexamphetamine ('speed') to stabilise metabolism."

"Perhaps all they need to do is stop drinking tap water first thing in the morning, says Dr. Brian Gulson, chief research scientist at the CSIRO Division of Exploration Geoscience. 'Tens of thousands of pregnant women and children in Australia are currently at risk of lead poisoning from toxic residues in their drinking water, 'Dr. Gulson warned a NSW parliamentary select committee on lead pollution in 1994, after announcing the results of a CSIRO study of the effects of plumbing systems on the lead content of drinking water."

"'The study, conducted at houses in the Sydney suburbs of Turramurra, Burwood, and Epping, and in Broken Hill for comparison , revealed dangerous lead levels in tap water which had been standing in the pipes for several hours – up to 12 times more than is considered 'safe' although, as the NHMRC points out, there is really no such thing as a safe lead level. "Safe in this context probably means it does not appear to be causing DETECTABLE harm. The levels were sometimes observed to be 32 times higher than the lead levels usually found in Australian Water Supplies."

"Remember that it took scientists 20 years to prove that inhaled asbestos caused cancer. We may wait just as long again to learn about its other properties. It's a risk many people are not prepared to take."

High Rise Lead

"Another problem peculiar to large offices is lead contamination in water left detained in pipelines during weekends and holidays. Some of the highest lead levels found during the Perth study were recorded in drinking water in high-rise buildings. There is no simple solution to this problem. Unlike household supplies, the volume of water necessary to flush all of the polluted water from the pipelines of a building fifteen or twenty storeys high makes flushing impractical."

"The only effective protection is the purification of all office drinking water or the provision of spring-water chillers, two options which are rapidly increasing in popularity."

Schools And Workplace Environments Are Now Starting To Install Filtered Drinking Water For Workers And Students

For people who went to school in the 50s and later, and beyond, you will remember the old school BUBBLERS as they called them. Unfortunately there are still many around in some schools. Memories of my childhood include our old school days when we had a giant thirst we had to put up with drinking water mostly hot from the bubblers on very hot days (hardly refreshing or cooling), plus fresh bottles of cows' milk, often times bottles would sit in the sun, and we pupils had to drink it hot; on a good day the milk would be given to us cold, early in the day, which was more refreshing.

I have noticed and it is good to observe that the better-off or private schools or those who are aware are installing filtered and temperature controlled and refreshing water fountains, also known as Acqua Fill, Water Refill Bottle Stations, but some schools are a bit slow catching up with water knowledge and installing the new technology, therefore the old bubblers are still around in some schools. Aqua Fill Stations are a step in the right direction to drinking healthy water at school.

Many businesses and industries are slowly catching up with clean drinking water and installing the Water Refill Bottle Stations which is a step in the right direction.

What Are School Students Drinking At Home

Okay, school students might drink from Water Refill Stations at school, but what are they drinking at home? What type of water (or other liquids) do these young people drink at home, such as unfiltered tap water or many types of soft drinks or cola, caffeinated and fizzy drinks or packaged fruit juices loaded with sugar?? Parents need to overhaul all drinking practices in the home.

There are still many people who stubbornly refuse to get home water filtering systems installed in their homes, some believing if they "boil" their tap water first and put it in the fridge to cool, it will remove the impurities. Unfortunately this method only gets rid of the bacteria, but doesn't remove the toxic chemicals like chlorine, fluoride and heavy metals, lead, pesticides, etc. There are also some people who don't want to outlay the money or mistakenly think that boiling tap water first removes all the impurities. Then there are those who are unaware of what they are drinking in tap water, or who simply do not want to install a home filtering water system, nor can they justify spending their money on something they deem to be unnecessary, but their priorities are in another direction and wouldn't think twice about buying an expensive coffee machine or an equally expensive wine collection.

To Drink From Plastic Bottles Or Other Types Of Drinkware

There are many people who drink bottled water today and it is quite acceptable, but I have an issue about carrying around water in a plastic bottle all day whilst you are out, especially if it is left in a motor vehicle and gets over-heated. Some bottled waters contain chemicals which when heated if left in the car or even out shopping can get over-heated and the plastic can leach into their drinking water. Taxi drivers and bus drivers take heed! It is advisable to avoid containers which contain PVC or BPA chemicals as they can contain a hormone disrupting chemical called bisphenol S (BPS). There are other alternative safe types of drinking containers such as small soft drink glass bottles or stainless steel flasks where the temperature can be controlled by the user, either room temperature, (room temperature can be cold in winter time) to warm or cold, according to the seasons, but alas drinking water should never be drunk cold, the reason being when it reaches the stomach, it has a cold effect on the internal organs, disrupting normal digestion.

I, myself prefer to drink water slightly warm, as it is much easier to drink; it seems to go down easier and is much more palatable, especially in the winter months. I also prefer to transfer my drinking water from my Reverse Osmosis home filter into a small soft drink glass bottle which can be used over and over again without any concerns; the taste is very refreshing, it never alters. Glass is a natural product and don't forget glass has been around a lot longer than plastic-ware, glass not having any health concerns. There could be breakages where children are concerned, so in that case a metal flask or other non-plastic container should be used. There are now plastic drink bottles available for children which are BPAs and BPS free. I also use a metal flask to transport water with me if I am going out for the whole day.

In relation to the above topic there are two articles worth reading – "BPA FREE SPORTS AND DRINKING BOTTLES" and "GREEN ECO LIVING PTY.LTD. IS BOTTLED WATER SAFER THAN TAP WATER" on line.

Another recent article written by Dr. Joseph Mercola about bottled water is also worth reading – MORE DECEPTION ABOUT BOTTLED WATER - DR. MERCOLA, retrieved AUG. 2015.

The above article is taken from Dr. Mercola's monthly newsletters where he mentions bottled water also and connections to many health conditions in women including ovarian toxicity. Could this be the reason there is an increased incidence of ovarian cancer? More research needs to be done.

In conclusion to this chapter, John Archer explains fully on pages 87, 88, 89, 90, 91,92 93 of the above book, the types and cost of Water filters available.

Although John Archer's book "The Water you Drink, how safe is it?" was published in 1996, Sydney Water quality is mostly unchanged, and some areas of Sydney I have tasted tap water which has a very noticeable taste of chlorine. People who are used to drinking tap water may not notice the chlorine taste, but people who are used to always drinking Reverse Osmosis home filtered water, can taste the difference straight away (ghastly).

If you are renovating and installing a new kitchen, I recommend installing either a ZIP Reverse Osmosis System where provision is made on the kitchen bench for an instant hot and cold water tap, or the newer model ISE RO System which involves a plumber drilling a small hole in the kitchen bench near the sink with filters under the sink, and both a hot and cold water spout is supplied thus providing instant hot or cold water as desired. This latter system (the RSE) takes up little space on the kitchen bench, also eliminating the need for a kettle or jug, therefore allowing space for other kitchen items.

For the ultimate in the latest water filtering information and professional service and expertise, I recommend and obtain all my water filtering products from "THE WATER SHOP" situated at 425 Miller Street, CAMMERAY, New South Wales and their other store at 342-350 Parramatta Rd, STANMORE, New South Wales.

Chapter 15

Too Much Pharmacology – Not Enough Naturopathy

Too much pharmacology, not enough naturopathy; what does it mean? From my perspective it means that when doctors finish their base medical degree, they have studied everything there is to know about pharmaceutical drugs, and which drugs help with certain illnesses, but UNFORTUNATELY they have not studied naturopathy, or very little of it. Naturopathy entails subjects like diet and Human Nutrition mainly, along with other associated health subjects which vary from course to course. It is important to note that it is rather IRONIC that the very subjects they fail to learn during their time at Medical School (which is diet and Nutrition) are the very subjects they SHOULD be studying so they can correctly advise their patients on which foods are good and which are not. The other sad irony is that the very people patients look up to and respect and ask for much needed dietary advice, (the Medical Profession) are the ones who have the LEAST training in those areas and so have the least dietary information for their patients. Ironies abound; the other sad irony is that doctors are also not trained properly in Bowel Health, ironically again the colon is one of the most important organs in the human body, yet it is one of the most neglected organs, and one which people know very little about. Bowel Health studies should be a subject so important and crucial to our general well-being, learning about the Gut and from where most diseases stem from. Current medical studies do not cover what is and what is not a good bowel motion or how often people should be having bowel motions.

Doctors Not Taught About Diet And Nutrition

Why aren't doctors taught about diet and nutrition? Doctors are grossly under-educated in these subjects and on many occasions more often than not, when patients ask their GPS or specialists what is a good diet, more often than not, are very vague or side-step the subject without a satisfactory answer. Is it because they haven't had the appropriate training in nutrition and dietary subjects and do not feel confident on that level? Is it also that because they have studied for 6 years plus, that they think that the subjects they have studied is all there is to know (pharmaceutical drugs and radical conventional orthodox treatment)? How wrong is that mentality?

With all due respects to the Medical Profession, when they enter Medical School and study to become a doctor, their Medical Degree hardly covers the studies of Diet and Nutrition, the current and grossly outdated amount of studyinvolved in Diet and Nutrition is between 6 – 20 hrs.(if that).

When I was first diagnosed with cancer I happened to speak to a young doctor (about 40) and I asked him how much nutritional study he had learned in his medical degree, he told me it was very little and wished he had learned much more and consequently couldn't confidently advise his patients on good nutrition as the subjects on Diet and Nutrition were not included in the Medical Degree curriculum, and he felt he needed much more knowledge in that direction.

Without my knowledge of naturopathy and wholistic diet and cures, I could never have survived my two life-threatening forms of cancer, namely Non-Hodgkin's Lymphoma and Stage 2 Cancer.

Doctors can't teach what they don't learn, and I think the whole Medical Studies curriculum needs to be overhauled so that when doctors finally finish their Medical Degree, along with post-graduate studies on Diet and Human Nutrition, they can enter it totally empowered and confidently know how to correctly advise their patients on diet and nutrition, but mainly from a wholistic approach as well as a scientific approach, thus saving more lives in the process.

Whilst I admire and appreciate all the obligatory lengthy study involved to become a doctor, and post-graduate studies to become Specialists, including all the wonderful life-saving operations and expert knowledge they possess when treating their patients. I question, however, their lack of important dietary knowledge and human nutrition they could pass on to their patients with extracurricular nutritional studies.

The Medical Profession Is Losing The Fight Against Cancer

Is the Medical Profession beholden to the Pharmaceutical Industry? Or does the Pharmaceutical Industry have a stranglehold on the Medical Profession? Is the Medical Profession pharmaceutically driven? Whatever the reason, post graduate courses on diet and nutrition must be included; things must change so that ALL doctors must learn about the fundamentals of diet and nutrition from a wholistic approach, and not just a scientific approach. Sadly Orthodox Medicine and Medical Profession in general is losing the fight against Cancer and until such time that doctors, that is GPs and Specialists alike, realise and study and admit that those two four-letter words, DIET AND FOOD have a strong correlation with cancer and other illnesses, there will NEVER be a successful long term natural cure for Cancer, without all the conventional, orthodox treatments with their horrendous side-effects, in many instances causing death.

It always breaks my heart every day when I hear of the thousands of people dying every day from cancer all over the world; it makes me feel very sad and gives me a feeling of helplessness when I know there is another way to fight it – a better way – a natural way, using food as medicine, but obviously people in the Medical Profession aren't interested in discussing healthy dietary regimens, consequently fewer people would get sick and then no-one connected to the Medical Profession would make much money out of it. What? All from eating a healthy diet? Yes, that's correct! If people knew how to eat healthily then they wouldn't need to see a doctor – there's no money in that!

'It's really very simple – a method through corrective or proper diet, without harmful drugs and without all the horrendous side-effects from poisonous chemotherapy and burns from radiation and sometimes radical invasive and sometimes unnecessary surgery.

It is at this point POST CANCER and after all the orthodox treatments have been exhausted, that doctors and associated physicians should advise cancer patients(and other patients with other illnesses to adopt what I call "the Biblical Diet" where they should eat large amounts of fruit and vegetables and salads and only drink plenty of filtered water and natural fluids, like green and herbal tea and fresh vegetable and fruit juices.

When the medical profession declares that a patient is CURED from cancer after the magic 5 year period, that is often not correct that it is cured forever. Cancers can and often do recur in some people after that 5 year period on many occasions where the cancer spreads to other organs in the body. In most cases patients are prescribed further harmful chemotherapy rendering the patient very very ill, losing their hair again and loosing too much weight, unable to eat because of their nauseousness and often over prescribing of radical orthodox treatments, consisting of large doses of chemotherapy and radiation, often causing death.

8-9 MILLION PEOPLE DIE ANNUALLY ALL OVER THE WORLD FROM CANCER

The Medical Profession is losing the fight against cancer as is evidenced by the staggering statistic of between 8 to 9 million DYING WORLDWIDE ANNUALLY from the disease, according to the World Health Organisation. And on top of the above frightening statistic, WHO predict that there will be a 70% increase in new cases of cancer worldwide in the next two decades, and those numbers will double. It is not known of course just how many people will die from the disease but be sure numbers will be high? Half of the people who have died from Cancer prematurely, should not have, dying way before their time, if only they'd been given correct dietary intervention advised by the Medical Profession.

COUNTRIES WHICH HAVE THE HIGHEST RATES OF CANCER

According to the Dana-Farber Cancer Institute, June 27th 2014, the countries with the highest rates of cancer surprisingly are: DENMARK, which ranks the highest, because of many people taking up smoking, high alcohol consumption and lack of exercise, and probably because of the Danish diet of pastries, cheeses and high carbohydrates. The second highest is FRANCE and thirdly, embarrassingly is

AUSTRALIA! Countries which have the lowest rates of cancer are several African countries, one reason being African people eat a mostly plant-based, vegetarian diet, MORE evidence that diet and cancer are connected. Another reason being they are not exposed to environmental chemicals like we are in the West.

The above information can be read in its entirety on" Dana Farber Cancer Institute Jan.27th 2014."

It breaks my heart when I hear of yet another person dying from Cancer prematurely, who if they had been given proper dietary advice in time could have prolonged their lives a lot longer. I have now seen so many people myself, friends and family who have died unnecessarily and prematurely from Cancer. In many instances many members of a family have been wiped out by Cancer WITHOUT ANY holistic dietary advice whatsoever given from orthodox trained conventional doctors. What a tragedy! Many young families today have lost babies and young children and parents and grandparents to cancer, some children losing their parents, who died very young and other children who similarly have lost their grandparents to cancer, and grow up never having known the love and care only parents and grandparents can bring.

Proper dietary advice could have helped to prolong their lives a lot longer. I more often than not get very annoyed when I hear people dying from cancer prematurely, not having a chance to fight it through a holistic approach with dietary means, only through radical conventional methods which often don't work and are so destructive to the body.

It makes my blood boil when I hear about doctors who know very little about food and the study of "diet and nutrition" and use phrases to tell people to "eat what they like" or "nothing causes cancer and there is no cure" I think "why don't they know? Why don't they know what I have read and researched for the last thirty years, by my extensive reading, and going to Health Seminars and consulting with many Health Professionals while I was suffering with arthritis and other ailments that I was determined to learn all about food and healthy nutrients?

Why don't they know what naturopaths and those health professionals who work in Alternative Medicine know and have known for decades that a healthy and detoxifying diet can and DOES shrink cancerous tumours? The Medical Profession SHOULD know! I think " get real". If I can cure my own two life-threatening cancers only eating healthy foods, and to reiterate the quote from Hippocrates that states "Let food be thy medicine and medicine be thy food". If it worked for me it can and does work for everyone else. What makes anyone else any different from me that they can't be cured? Similarly other killer diseases like Diabetes, Multiple Sclerosis, Motor-Neuron disease and Parkinson's disease and Alzheimer's and other serious illnesses can be helped or cured or even eradicated completely, using a dietary approach, but they are never given a chance or explored by orthodox medicine.

How much longer must this VITAL lack of dietary and nutritional knowledge within orthodox medicine be kept from the public? It is long overdue that Doctors in the Medical profession learn all about proper dietary studies and the wider community MUST be informed! This scepticism and dogmatic attitude towards diet and alternative therapies within Orthodox Medicine requires an overhaul and needs to change very soon.

Just think – such a simple factor like healthy eating and corrective diet can have a huge impact on the state of our health and longevity!

Hospitals Are Over-Crowded

There are many many hospitals and hospices all over the world, many of them seem to be overcrowded and overflowing with sick patients. In most hospitals there seems to be a shortage of beds and staff, one reason being the increasing numbers of sick and ailing people. Hospital and medical staff can't seem to keep up with the demands for beds despite new hospitals being built all the time.

Imagine this hypothetical scenario - where hospitals and doctors pushed proper dietary advice instead of over-prescribing pills? While we're discussing proper dietary advice, hospital food in general is not the healthiest food that is served to patients. Also the food served in many childrens' hospitals leaves a lot to be desired; that needs to be addressed as well.

DIETARY ADVICE NOT PILLS

If patients were given correct dietary advice in the beginning of a person's illness, or after operations, possibly preventing them from even having the need to be admitted to hospital in the first place, with patients possibly being cured from their illnesses. The consequences would be that more beds would be available for hospital patients, and then possibly alleviating the need to build more hospitals, thus lightening the load on the Health System and saving Governments millions of dollars. The flow-on effect from that would be the Pharmaceutical Companies, Pharmacies and associated Medicos may not make the billions of dollars they already make. I can't see that happening anytime soon!

Many Patients Are Over Medicated

Why is it that doctors and hospital nurses alike in hospitals push pharmaceutical drugs onto patients whether they need them or not. It would be better if doctors were to discuss with the patient if some of these drugs can be eliminated as they can be expensive and a great burden to their patients and may not be necessary. By the same token, patients need to ask their doctors themselves if some of their medications can be reduced or eliminated altogether. Many of the drugs used in hospitals can disrupt sleep patterns, or cause other serious side-effects. Doctors and Medical hospital staff need to confer together with all patients, regardless of their ailments or their diseases, serious or otherwise, to apply the brakes on too many medications as too many hospital patients today are seriously over-medicated, which is expensive and a great burden on the health system, often causing many serious side-effects to the patients. Why is this happening? Do hospitals and the Medical Profession have another agenda? Are they pharmaceutically driven? Or are they just putting profit before patients' health.

This over-medication does not only take place in hospitals, there are many doctors' other outpatients who consult their doctors at their surgeries or in a Medical Centre setting, who are also over-medicated. I have heard of some patients who take up to 20 different medications a day for their ailments and that is just the tip of the iceberg. Many of those medications are not necessary and over-medication can cause doctors' patients more serious health concerns, with worrying side-effects, not to mention the cost of such medications. Many of these patients are elderly and could be well-advised by their doctors to adopt a healthy diet and lifestyle, with the aim of reducing or completely eliminating their medications altogether, along with considerable monetary savings.

There needs to be greater scrutiny into all patients' medications, if some of them can be eliminated, whether they are hospital patients or otherwise.

Cancer Is Big Business

Cancer is a multi-billion dollar industry and there are a lot of people making a lot of money from it. Where do all the billions of dollars raised in the name of "Cancer Research" go? I know a good chunk of it goes into employing more nurses in chemotherapy wards to administer chemo treatment. Is that research?? Hardly! The public have been promised a cure that is "just around the corner" yet there doesn't seem to be any "major breakthroughs" yet. The Medical Profession is no further advanced in finding a cure for Cancer than they were 50 years ago.

Cancer charities all over the world are getting richer and richer from donations from the wider community in general. Billions of dollars have been raised from donations from the public (that's you and me) and the public is getting poorer and poorer from those donations, plus the financial burden from their cancer treatments, but more importantly from the lack of real health information to heal their cancers and other ailments sadly lacking from most sections of the Medical Profession.

WHERE IS THAT ELUSIVE CURE FOR CANCER?

The Medical Profession and scientists alike are searching for that elusive, so called "miracle drug" to cure cancer. Will they ever discover it? Are they searching too hard for a complicated explanation or rare gene for a cancer cure, focusing too much on genes or hereditary factors? Perhaps the answer may lie right under their noses or rather in the Gut? We need to go back to nature and eat the diet God intended us to eat as explained in Chapter 1 and live like the people did in Ancient Times and adopt "The Biblical Diet" that is eating the foods from God's Garden, consisting of large quantities of fresh fruit and vegetables, and drinking lots of filtered water. Water was pure in those times, not like todays drinking water which is filled with chemicals.

I would like to suggest that the above answers are helping to prevent and heal cancer and all other serious life-threatening diseases as already mentioned like Parkinsons, Multiple Sclerosis, Motor Neuron Disease, even Alzheimers Disease, etc. which, incidentally, Orthodox Medicine states that there are no known medical cures for the above illnesses. What about proper dietary intervention, naturally, without medication with all its serious side-effects?

My own rapid Cancer cure is a testimony in itself for using food as medicine, when in October this year, at time of writing (October, 20015) I was declared "5 years cancer-free" by my Cancer Specialist. These unique results were by my adherence to a natural diet and lifestyle, with minimal orthodox treatment.

Cancer Is A Cash Cow

Cancer is a cash cow and let me mention just a few occupations who are directly or indirectly making money from Cancer. Firstly there are the Pharmaceutical Companies (Big Pharma), then there are all pharmacies and their associated employees. Recent reports expose many hospital car parks which are run by large multinational firms, which are raking in millions of dollars from vulnerable friends and relatives visiting sick or cancer patients undergoing short or long term chemotherapy, the financial cost being exorbitant for the above people who have to pay for extended parking by the hour.

Lets move on – there are the Radiographers, Haematologists, and the many staff in Radiation Oncology Departments in large hospitals, the Surgical Oncologists, Radiation Oncologists, Medical Oncologists, Paediatric Oncologists, Integrative Oncologists, Gynaecological Oncologists, Dieticians, Radiation Oncology Nurses of Allied Health, Medical Physicists, Psychologists, and other doctors and surgeons who may be associated with cancer. There are Patient Care Technicians, Social Workers, Clinical Office Assistants, Medical Dosimetrists, Occupational Therapists, Physiotherapists and the Palliative Care consultants, and all the doctors, nurses and other people who work in the Palliative Care Hospitals, Childrens' Hospitals, and hospitals in general. Don't forget the many nurses who administer chemotherapy or radiation or work in Cancer Wards in the many, many hospitals. Then you have the surgeons, general surgeons, plastic surgeons who perform mastectomies and then later on perform breast reconstruction after the aftermath of mastectomies. It indicates to me that there seems to be a different kind of Specialist Surgeon for the many types of Cancers invading the population. That in itself must create more jobs?

Let us not forget the Wig Industry – most people who have cancer treatment, that is chemotherapy/ and or radiation more often than not lose their hair and have to buy a wig as all their hair falls out. There is also the scarf and hat industry, where many people who may not want to, or can afford a wig, buy scarves and hats.

The Funeral Industry Is Huge

Let us not forget to mention the Funeral Industry and whose associated occupations are profiting from Cancer. They are the Funeral Parlours, Casket Builders, the Crematoriums, and their employees, the Stone Masons, florists, the Caterers who provide Wakes after the Funeral Services at the cemeteries. The Grave Diggers and many of the other people who are connected to the Funeral Industry who have gone unmentioned here and who are connected in some way to the DEATH INDUSTRY or other relevant occupations. There are thousands of people feeding off the "cash cow" and that cash cow is CANCER.

FOOD FOR THOUGHT

Whilst there is cancer in our society there will ALWAYS be employment for the above professions and occupations. In a world WITHOUT cancer there would be MASS unemployment.

DAISY LUTHER, A FREELANCE WRITER, EDITOR, ACTIVIST AND BLOGGER, GIVES HER REVELATIONS BELOW ON CANCER DATED Dec. 10th 2013: THE ORGANIC PREPPER
MAKING A KILLING WITH CANCER $A124.6 BILLION DOLLAR INDUSTRY

"There will never be a "cure" brought to market because there just isn't enough profit in eradicating the disease entirely.
        "There will never be a governing body that protects consumers from being subjected to known carcinogens, because that too will stop the cash from rolling in. A great deal of research is covered up and many potential cures are ignored and discredited because there is far more money in perpetuating illness than in curing it".
        "In 2012, the reported spending on cancer treatment was 124.6 million dollars. BLOOD MONEY!

The above article can be read in its entirety on the above website. "ALL HEALTH, DEC,2013 THE ORGANIC PREPPER".

A Change Is In Sight

In relation to medical students learning about the subjects of Diet and Nutrition, a change is in sight.

Due to increased consumer demands, more Australian GPs and physicians and other allied health professionals are now undertaking or who have already completed further studies in Alternative Medicine on top of their base of clinical or Hospital based studies.

I believe there is a 3 year Post Graduate course in Diet and Nutrition that Medical Students can undertake on top of their base Medical Degree. The base Degree is about 6 years and the Post Graduate course of Complimentary and Integrative Medicine is about another three years. These courses vary from university to university and country to country. Many medical students may not want to continue studying after their Base Medical Course of 6 years and do a minimum of 3 more years of post-graduate study, but it is worth it to finish their studies with the extra three years CAIM tagged onto their base Medical Degree, with a complete knowledge of disease through scientific Pharmacology AND Naturopathy and Nutrition, plus the added knowledge of a holistic approach to illness through correct diet and nutrition, and with a sense of empowerment. These post graduate courses in my mind should be compulsory and for all medical students entering universities from now on. It would also be advisable for "old school" doctors and doctors who have been in the profession for many years to undertake naturopathic and post graduate studies.

These postgraduate courses in Complimentary and Integrative Medicine are not happening often or quick enough for me, as there are still too many old school doctors who have learned medicine the old way, and who adamantly believe that diet and nutrition DO NOT have any correlation with cancer and other diseases. In fact there are many GPs and specialists alike who when presented with patients who have cured their cancers with dietary or natural methods, ignore, deny, scoff at, suppress or even ridicule a dietary or alternate approach to fighting cancer.

There are some patients who even dare to suggest to their doctors that healthy diets might help with cancer who are met with hostility and intimidation by the Medical Profession. That is because they have no understanding of the rudiments of foods. And then there are also those people who work in the field of conventional and scientific mainstream medicine and scientific naysayers. The doomsayers and sceptics alike will say my cancer cure was anecdotal evidence, a one-off, a fluke, just good luck, and that my two cancers were TREATABLE, which means that they weren't serious, and there was no scientific evidence or scientifically proven explanation for my CURE.

My answer to these people is this: "well try and scientifically DISPROVE my cancer cure" Many dismiss alternate therapies as "quackery" Many of them state adamantly that cancer cannot be prevented or even cured, saying that "there is no known cause for cancer and no known natural alternative cure", saying that cancer patients have just had "bad luck", and could possibly or probably die. Why do doctors continue to say that? Why do they think that way? Is it because they feel threatened that their livelihood might be in jeopardy, or is it that they think because they have studied for six years plus that their Medical Degree is almost worthless if diet were the key to most diseases? Doctors prefer on the other hand to prescribe what they have been trained for, to recommend orthodox, conventional and radical medical treatments such as chemotherapy, which is a poison to the body and radiation which can cause serious burns to the patient, and often times surgeons perform radical and unnecessary invasive surgery, cutting out organs or mutilating limbs. Chemotherapy and radiation treatment can and does leave patients very sick, with nausea, vomiting and diarrhoea, confined to bed and unable to function on a day-to-day basis, as I can attest to.. Chemotherapy may kill cancer cells but it also destroys good cells doing untold damage.

Whilst I understand patients may need lifesaving drugs I think they are sometimes OVER-PRESCRIBED. The above horrendous symptoms most often continue and worsen when cancer patients have to endure more and more chemotherapy and radiation later on as the cancer spreads to other organs. At this point death is tragically inevitable to these poor patients. This mentality is incorrect, and from my perspective, in view of the fact that I cured my own two life-threatening cancers with a minimum of orthodox treatment but with a MAXIMUM of diet and nutrition therapy. There are also many books which have been written by other cancer survivors, who adopted a healthy dietary approach to their illnesses, and have survived many years post cancer, but often do not get recognised by the Medical Profession.

Orthodox Treatments Are Sometimes Necessary

I am not totally undermining orthodox medicine or treatments in any way, or the Medical Profession, because sometimes it may be necessary to undergo a minimum of conventional treatments for cancer, if the disease is life-threatening, such as was the case in my instance where I was told I wouldn't survive cancer without radical chemotherapy which left me very very ill and lost all my hair, even though I had the lowest minimum dose of chemo recommended by my Specialist which was JUST 6 treatments.

The issue I have with chemotherapy and radiation is when a patient has already had about six bouts of chemotherapy and then the cancer may have spread, and treatment hasn't worked, then the patient is coerced into having many more multiple bouts of POISONOUS chemotherapy and radiation, thus rendering the patient unable to function in everyday life and being very very sick. After all this shocking treatment the patient still has not improved and the cancer flourishes, and on many occasions the patient still DOES NOT survive their cancers, short-term or long-term, despite having to endure more orthodox treatments. These scenarios I don't like nor can I understand. To put cancer patients through all the misery, pain and nausea, along with a feeling of helplessness, putting more poison from orthodox chemotherapy and burns from radiation into their bodies, and at great financial burden, seems futile and unnecessary.

In my opinion, when a patient is first diagnosed with cancer, and later after undergoing all radical orthodox methods of treatment, chemo and or radiation, or surgery, and when all treatments have been exhausted, it is at THAT point, POST cancer treatment where diet, lifestyle and nutritional advice should be immediately recommended to the oncology patient, by their Specialists, thus giving them at least a better chance of survival and beating their cancer. More often than not there is NO amount of proper dietary advice given. Ironically it is "the missing link for survival".

CANCER PATIENTS TRAVEL OVERSEAS FOR CURES

There are many people afflicted with cancer, who after exhausting all methods of orthodox mainstream methods of treatment, are recommended or decide for themselves, to travel to overseas countries like America, or Europe, to seek out other methods of cancer cures, searching for that elusive answer. Many have had Stem-cell treatment and other means of treatments. Stem cell treatment is only in its infancy and has not had a chance to see if it works long-term. Some cancer patients have undergone treatment overseas but often times it has not worked because dietary measures are seldom recommended. In those instances the long distances travelled, can take a toll on the body of the ailing cancer patient, rendering that course of treatment futile.

Cancer strikes people from all walks of life; it doesn't discriminate. It strikes people from all professions and occupations, nationalities and cultures. Doctors do not escape cancer either; they also have high rates of cancer themselves as well as their loved ones, which must be devastating and disheartening when you would think they would have some idea as to how to prevent the aftermath of horrible side-effects from cancer treatment and possibly death.

As far as I am concerned, cancer patients need not have to travel overseas, when the treatment should start in one's own back yard, right here in Australia, or their own country, where ever that may be, in our own kitchens, a place where all miracles take place, or should take place, by spending time in the kitchen by preparing life-giving foods and lots of fluids in a healthy manner.

Dietician Or Naturopath?

Most hospital dieticians have completed studies at university from a scientific point of view and are not trained to look at the "big picture" when treating a patient. They are usually Accredited Practising Dieticians (ACP) but not Nutritionists or Naturopaths. The Medical Profession doesn't agree to strict diets being prescribed, where certain foods or drinks are not recommended to the cancer patient. This method of treatment is not recommended or accepted by conventional nutritional science based medicine. Hospital dieticians think any calories are good calories, and often prescribe foods that are just empty calories to their patients. They often tell patients to sometimes eat much of what they desire, even fatty ice-cream, dairy foods, sometimes rich foods which may be banned by a naturopath. Doctors similarly often wrongly advise cancer patients to eat anything which helps to put weight on, whether it be fast food or fattening unhealthy foods, in fact any foods which they think will aid in putting the weight back on, which they have drastically lost due to the ravages of their cancer treatment.

I believe there are now Integrative Dieticians and Integrative Doctors appearing in some hospitals in America and they are now starting to appear in Australian Hospitals, I hope, which will be a step in the right direction.

In my case I never suffered as a result of restricting certain foods, but was able to eat many other nourishing foods and drinks which aided my rapid cure by detoxifying the body in a healthy manner. When I set about fighting my two life-threatening cancers, I initially restricted certain foods such as meat, dairy and gluten-free foods, sweets and chocolates. Certain foods were also restricted (there is more information on my dietary regime in the following chapter) and it was only due to the many years of research I have undertaken and diligence and focus on detoxifying and ridding my body of the two cancers that I happily succeeded. At the time of writing, I continue to do so as I pass the Magic five year mark, since my initial diagnosis and have now been declared "cancer- free" by my Cancer Specialist.

Naturopaths Look At The Bigger Picture

Qualified naturopaths on the other hand are fully qualified nutritionists, medical herbalists, and often homeopaths and also iridologists, who are trained to look at all aspects of diet and nutrition from a holistic point of view, including extensive studies of Bowel Health. They are however not recognised by the Medical Profession. It is therefore up to the patient to decide which health professional they choose to consult, either a dietician or a naturopath, or even a Complimentary and Integrative Dietician or Doctor when suffering from Cancer, Diabetes or other serious illnesses. When choosing your health professional, choose carefully and choose someone who will look at the "bigger picture" from a holistic point of view, as people need to know ALL options, holistic as well as scientific, then it will be easier to decide which avenues to embark on.

Chinese Medicine Is Useful

Practitioners who study Chinese Medicine are trained from a holistic approach and apply diet, Chinese herbs, massage, acupuncture, meditation, and other modalities and also from a spiritual point of view in their treatment. These treatments have been known to be successful for many cancer patients and other patients with serious ailments.

Until such time that ALL doctors learn about the all important fundamentals of diet and nutrition, it may be necessary for people to undertake Health courses themselves and read up on all the Health magazines and informative books about Cancer and health for their own well-being.

In conclusion, I even heard one day on a medical programme on American television, a doctor say that the Medical Textbooks should be re-written, worldwide, ensuring that Medical Students can learn with extensive and comprehensive studies on diet and nutrition, as current Medical Studies are outdated and archaic and do not relate to today's world in the 21st century. To quote the exact words of the above doctor she said "things must change."

Chapter 16

My Health Tips To Combat Cancer

To combat cancer or other illnesses it is important to note that there is no short cut to curing illnesses, especially cancer. There needs to be a lot of kitchen action that means spending a bit of time preparing meals like shopping for vegetables and healthy foods, food preparation, cutting and chopping up fresh ingredients for salads, and vegetables and cooking nutritious meals. For those folk who don't like cooking or are kitchen-shy or can't cook, or do not want to spend time in the kitchen, I am afraid there is no hope for them as there are no short-cuts to good health or healthy eating or combating illnesses like cancer and other diseases. If the non-kitchen participants and apron-haters can overcome their dislike for kitchen duties and try to get involved in trying healthy recipes, they will most likely gain more confidence with their cooking skills, giving them a sense of empowerment, and then they will start to feel better; to do so can bring an exhilarating feeling of well-being, good health and high energy, they may then want to go onto doing more and more home cooking with natural foods, and experiment cooking with foods they haven't tried before.

Dining Out Can Be Tricky

Eating take away foods or dining at restaurants on a regular basis is not recommended. It should only happen as a treat may be once a week or fortnight, and then choosing something rather healthy such as Asian or vegetarian or healthy seafood. Dining out at restaurants can be tricky as there are many additives such as MSG contained in Asian cuisine, and an overuse of salt and sugar in some sauces. Dining at other restaurants can be tricky too where other unhealthy additives such as butter and cream along with too much salt are added to enhance the flavour of the dishes. Eating a home-cooked meal is always the BEST option because YOU KNOW what goes in it.

On Juice Extractors

Owning a juice extractor is an appliance that is necessary to fight cancer and just to keep healthy. There are many brands on the market and it can be confusing choosing the right one. From my own experience it is better to invest in a good juicer rather than buying a cheaper regular juicer. When I purchased my first juicer thirty five years ago I purchased a regular juicer which didn't last long, then I bought four more cheap regular juicers which didn't last long either, and then I finally learnt the obvious lesson that often times you get what you pay for, and then bought a "Champion" brand. I found out the hard way that it was false economy buying certain regular juicers. When choosing a juicer it should be the non-centrifugal type which means they don't get overheated and vitamins and fibre aren't destroyed; vitamins are left intact. The opposite happens when a centrifugal type is used (regular juicers) it means that when machines get over-heated, so do the vegetables being juiced, heat up thus limiting efficacy of vitamins and fibre content and effectiveness. Another tip to remember is juice should always be juice NOT a smoothie, as pure juice is often more detoxifying than a thick smoothie, which sometimes contain sugar-laden ingredients, which lack fibre and cause weight gain. The Champion is a non-centrifugal brand and I can say I have had it for thirty years and it is still going strong. Another advantage of owning a Champion Juicer is that it comes with an easily adjusted attachment which makes delicious nut spreads.

The Champion is not available in retail stores but can be purchased from the Importers & Distributors of the Champion Juicer at the address below. When juicer attachments wear out they can also be purchased from the phone no. below. The juicer costs around $550.00 AUD. Their address is: CHAMPION JUICER SALES OF AUSTRALIA, 121 Ramsay Terrace, BORDERTOWN. 5268. SOUTH AUSTRALIA. Phone No. is 1800 033 866.

FOOD STORAGE

Don't store food in plastic containers in the refrigerator, except food can be stored in plastic containers and kept in the freezer. Use only glass or earthenware bowls (ceramic) for the fridge, and when storing salads. Don't store cakes or biscuits in plastic containers or plastic jars either. Use only glass jars or tin containers. Cakes and slices can be stored in the freezer section of the refrigerator and taken out when needed. They can keep for several months if wrapped and sealed well, in foil and then in a plastic bag.

Lifestyle

Don'ts

- Avoid alcohol
- Don't use drugs such as marijuana, cocaine, heroin or ice, etc.
- Don't smoke

Do

- Go for a daily walk, and/or do weight-bearing exercises like lifting light weights.
- Do light gym work or Pilates, or yoga once or twice a week.
- Go for a swim or attend aqua aerobic or hydrotherapy classes, once or twice a week.
- Attend dance classes.
- Indulge in activities that are relaxing.
- Try to keep active.

The above exercises should only be done under a Doctor's supervision.

- Try to get 8 hrs. sleep nightly

Diet

Foods to avoid in combating cancer

- Don't eat a high animal protein diet
- Don't eat hamburgers or deep fried foods
- Avoid high fat dairy foods, such as feta cheese, hard or salty cheeses, yoghurts which contain sugar, milk, coconut milk or ice cream, margarines, but a minimum of butter on crackers or bread. (Calcium can be obtained from other foods)
- Avoid cakes, pastries, muffins, sweet biscuits, and highly salted crackers, chocolates and lollies.
- Don't eat white flour products that are white rice, pre-cooked rice, regular pasta, lasagne, etc. white bread, pizza, potato crisps and all other snack foods or instant meals from the supermarket.
- Avoid all cured and processed meats, ham, corned beef, pastrami, salami, mortadella, cabanossi, frankfurts, prosciutto, smoked or processed meats like chicken or turkey, etc. because of salt and chemical content.

- Avoid all smoked or cured fish such as salmon, trout, oysters, etc.
- Avoid fish containing mercury such as sword fish, tuna, ling, deep sea fish, cod or snapper, etc.
- Avoid all crustaceans (shellfish) prawns, shrimps, lobster, crabs, scallops, Balmain bugs, oysters, etc. as they contain cholesterol, high salt, and are the scavengers of the sea, and are hard to digest. Not widely publicised also is the fact that crustaceans, if eaten regularly can and do cause allergies and other serious ailments in many people.
- Restrict vegetables from the Nightshade and Solanaceae family, eggplants, capsicums, tomatoes and potatoes because of their high acidity. (which also aggravate arthritis conditions)
- Restrict beans, peas and corn, the latter can cause allergic reaction or hard to digest.
- Avoid peanuts, raw and roasted as they contain aflatoxin which is harmful to the body and can cause allergies and anaphalaxis.
- Avoid highly salted foods and such as olives, anchovies, capers, sundried tomatoes, pickled vegetables, and condiments like mustard, and all bottled sauces, and white and brown and balsamic vinegar. (high acidity and fermented) stock cubes with MSG.
- Avoid most canned goods, soups, juices and packaged and frozen foods and TV dinners as they contain a lot of salt or sugar and preservatives.

- Don't eat starchy soups such as pumpkin, potato or parsnip, or soups with cream as they are hard to digest.
- Cut out or restrict all salt as it holds fluid in the body and is partly responsible for high blood pressure.
- Don't use any type of vinegar including balsamic, except apple cider vinegar (use lemon juice instead)
- Use Himalayan Crystal Salt sparingly if necessary.
- Restrict pepper as it is inflammatory, occasionally using cayenne pepper, occasionally, and go easy on spices as they are hard on the body.
- Restrict bananas, mangoes, as they are heavy and hard to digest, restrict oranges and mandarins for their acidity.
- Restrict grapes and strawberries and other berries if people are prone to any form of arthritis, as they are very acidic.

Drinks to avoid

- Coffee
- Tea
- Tap water
- Bottled water
- Alcohol or spirits
- Bottled or packaged fruit juices (for their high sugar content)
- Tomato juice (acidic)

- All soft drinks
- Caffeinated drinks
- Diet soft drinks
- Milk
- Some fattening smoothies

Well, you will say "what's left" PLENTY!

Note. Do not take fright or be turned off with the above list; it is a guide only, which should be adhered to only in the initial stages of ill health, but once health is restored slight relaxation of the above foods can be resumed. Now for the DO EATS:

On microwave use

- Cook ALL meals in a regular oven and hotplates or upright ranges.
- Restrict microwave oven use; use for occasional re-heating, only as a back-up when absolutely necessary.
- Don't store food in plastic ware in refrigerator or in cupboards or pantry, to avoid chemicals in same as plastic containers change the taste of food for the worst because of the chemical content. However food can be stored in plasticware in the freezer section of the refrigerator.
- Use instead earthenware, ceramic or glassware, or Pyrex bowls and jars and bottles to store foods in refrigerators or pantries. It will be noticeable that storing food in the above materials ensures that the taste of food is not affected and all foods

stored this way will obviously keep much longer and taste much better than if using plastic-ware.

Do eat

- Eat only small quantities of lean meat (organic where possible) once a week
- Do eat small amounts of organic or free-range chicken or turkey once a week.
- Do eat vegetarian patties or falafels occasionally with a large salad.
- Do eat legumes e.g. lentils, chick peas in moderation, as they have a protein inhibitor, so can be hard to digest for some people.
- Do eat in moderation, almonds, walnuts, brazil nuts or cashews, (preferably raw) or roasted unsalted.
- Do eat fresh salmon or ocean trout 2 or 3 times a week.
- Do eat white fish with bones (flathead, bream, whiting, etc.) as some fish with bones do not contain mercury and are easier to digest.
- Do eat eggs in moderation (two boiled eggs a week) or an omelette or vegetable quiche once a week
- Do eat home-made soups most nights as an entrée or a main meal, made from fresh produce (made with vegetables or legumes) as the RIGHT soups contain fibre and health-giving nutrients, which I see as a necessary food to prevent or fight disease.

Limit soups such as pumpkin and root vegetables as they are high in starch and hard to digest for some people.

When cooking soup make two or more different varieties in batches, simmering at the same time, then cool and freeze in meal-size containers for later use. This method gives more variety so a different soup can be eaten on alternate evenings.

- Do eat in unlimited amounts all vegetables from the brassica family of cruciferous vegetables which are: broccoli, broccolini, cauliflower, brussell sprouts, cabbage (hard variety), red cabbage, which has more anti-oxidants, Chinese cabbage, Chinese broccoli. Most leafy greens are detoxifying.

- Eat vegetables which contain the bitter element like globe artichokes, endive, chicory, radicchio etc.. These foods stimulate the liver which accelerate toxin removal, speeding up the detoxifying process which takes place in the intestines.

- Do eat in unlimited amounts brown onions, Spanish onions, garlic, leeks, chillies, ginger root, turmeric root, lemon grass, galangal (detoxifying)

- The good news on onions: onions contain folate, Vitamin B1, Vitamin C, Vitamin B6, dietary fibre, phosphorus and copper.

- A cooking tip for this underrated vegetable is to cook up a pan of lightly fried onions to go with the evening meal. I find it to be one of the best cleansing vegetables around.

- Do eat liberal amounts of all herbs such as FRESH parsley, coriander or cilantro, fresh rosemary, oregano, fresh and dried, fresh basil, fresh mint, fresh thyme, fresh lemon thyme, fresh sage, fresh dill, fresh chives, fresh and dried bay leaves.

- Try to eat the above herbs for flavouring food rather than salt.
- Do eat in large amounts all FRESH salad vegetables like cos or romaine lettuce, all other lettuces, celery, cucumbers, fennel, raw beetroot salads, and cooked beetroot etc. Eat organic produce where possible.
- Do eat (when in season) sliced raw fennel with lunch or dinner for good digestion.
- Do snack on carrot and celery sticks and which also can be eaten with meals for good digestion. These vegetables can be transported whilst shopping and can accompany a meal if dining out.
- Do eat kumera, potatoes, and pumpkin in moderation.
- Eat 1 slice gluten-free bread or heavy dark rye sourdough daily in moderation (available from health food stores) or buckwheat or rice bread which is gluten-free.
- Eat gluten-free crispbreads and those with a low salt content. Orgran Brand.
- Eat only brown rice and gluten-free spaghetti (Orgran and Buontempo are good brands and my favourite, which has all the allergens removed).

Fruits

- Do eat all the melons, watermelon, rockmelon, variations of honey-dew, apples, pears, paw-paw, papaya, persimmons, fuju fruit, when in season, autumn and winter, kiwi fruit, (gold variety are less acidic than green ones) grapefruit, tropical pineapples, cherries, , all stone fruit, tropical pineapples, mandarins in moderation, avocados, lemons and limes(are acidic, but which when eaten, become alkaline in the body)

Do drink

- Drink filtered water only (not cold) should be drunk slightly warm or room temperature. Drink 6-8 glasses of water daily, plus 1 vegetable juice and 1 mug green tea and 1 mug herbal tea (9 drinks in total)
- Drink fresh fruit and vegetable juices (one daily)
- It is important to drink the above fluids as they help to flush the kidneys (good kidney health) and liver function and rid the intestines of unwanted waste matter.
- Drink superior quality loose leaf green tea such as Oolong
- Drink herbal teas
- Drink hot water with slices of fresh ginger root allowed to brew
- Drink lime, SODA (not lemonade) and bitters (optional) when dining out (in moderation)

Below is my eating pattern which I follow to this day in combating cancer as it has been very helpful in detoxifying the digestive system, also energising and giving clarity of mind and a sense of wellbeing.

Breakfast

On rising
- 2 tablespoons aloe vera juice
- 2x 200 ml. glasses of warm filtered water, with a small squeeze of FRESH lemon juice, one after the other
- 1 glass vegetable juice, freshly made from the following:
- 1 medium carrot roughly chopped, unpeeled
- 1 celery stalk cut in pieces
- 1 piece fresh ginger root about 1 ½ inches
- ½ small beetroot washed, peeled and top removed and cut in small pieces
- 3 small chunks red or HARD white cabbage
- ¼ large or ½ small granny smith apple cut up and skin on

The above juice yields 1x200mls. glass of vegie and fruit juice. This is followed by:

- 1 serve watermelon and ½ or ¼ granny smith apple.
- 1 more 1x200 ml. glass warm water with a small squeeze of lemon juice.

- 1 slice gluten-free bread or dark rye bread baked or toasted topped with guacamole or tahini dip (recipes below) or homemade almond butter and a small spread butter.
- Buy dark rye sour dough bread or gluten-free bread, slice, freeze and take out one slice at a time from the freezer as needed. This bread tastes best when baked rather than toasted.
- 1 mug superior quality green tea like Oolong made with 1 teaspoon loose leaves and brewed for 5 mins. in a teapot (leaves can be used again)

TIPS. Oolong loose-leaf tea can be purchased from most Specialty Tea Shops.

- Also at breakfast time I take liquid fish oil and Bowel Probiotic capsules and Vitamin D3 (if needed) and a COQ10 tablet for heart health.

Mid-Morning

1x 200ml. glass water with three or four nuts, roasted or raw, and unsalted, almonds, walnuts, or Brazil nuts

Lunch

A large green salad comprising cos or romaine lettuce, rocket or arugula, radicchio,(Italian red lettuce) sliced cucumber, sliced celery, chopped mint, dressed in extra virgin olive oil and fresh lemon juice (never vinegar, as it very acidic) with one hardboiled egg, OR 2 thin slices of low salt cheese, OR an egg omelette made with grated zucchini, OR a small .piece pan fried or baked salmon or ocean trout OR a vegetable patty or falafel or several slices avocado and salad eaten with gluten-free crackers.

NOTE. All of the above proteins should be eaten with a large salad.

Recipes for salads to follow in next chapter.

2.00pm

- 1 glass water and small amount nuts

3.30pm

- 1 small serve of fruit, either kiwi gold, apple, pear, paw paw, pineapple, fuju fruit, mandarin

4.30pm

- 1 mug herbal or green tea
- 1 or 2 gluten-free crackers with either guacamole, tahini dip or almond spread

DINNER Eaten between 6-7.00pm

- 1 small bowl soup

- Bean stew or casserole of veal chops or lamb chops or lamb cutlets or organic free-range chicken or salmon or ocean trout or white fish with bones (bream or whiting or flathead). Team these proteins with boiled and mashed swede or carrots and piles of green leafy vegetables (as listed above)

OR

- Rice pilaf, or gluten-free spaghetti with pasta sauce with lots of leafy green vegetables

ALSO

- For dinner eat a coleslaw daily AND a Spanish onion salad along with the above animal protein and vegetables, OR starch meal of rice, pasta or starch vegetables such as pumpkin or kumera.
- Two salads a day should be eaten, one green for lunch and coleslaw for dinner, or vice versa.

After-Dinner Fruit

- Wait 2 hours
- 8.30pm
- 1 serve of any of the allowable fruits

Bedtime

- Best times to turn in - between 9.30pm and 10.30pm
- Just before retiring - 1 glass warm water with squeeze lemon juice or ¼ teas. medicinal turmeric (to strengthen the immune system and detox. the digestive system) in a glass of warm water

Sweet Dreams

- Recipes to follow in the last half of the book

Lunchtime Meal Suggestions

- 1 boiled egg with beetroot salad, large green salad, and slices of avocado and some gluten-free crispbreads OR 1 slice healthy bread
- 1 egg omelette with 1 tbls. grated zucchini and small amount Spanish onion sliced finely, and all of the above salads with crispbreads OR
- 1 small piece butterflied fresh salmon or ocean trout about 150g with the above salads with crispbreads OR
- 2 thin pieces cheese with low salt and vegetarian enzymes with the above salads with crispbreads OR
- Vegetarian or lentil patties or falafels or vegetarian pasties or healthy quiche with the above salads and crispbreads.

- Take salads from refrigerator ½ hr- 1hr. before eating (depending on the time of the year) as they are not as cold to eat, this tip makes salads more palatable.

The above meal ideas can be rotated to give some variation.

RECIPES

Most of the recipes in this book are wheat-free, yeast-free, gluten-free, dairy-free, egg- free and free of artificial preservatives, and created by myself. I hope you will enjoy preparing and eating them.

Tahini Dip

- 2 heaped. tbls. tahini
- 2 tbls. fresh lemon juice
- 1 tbls. chopped chives
- 2 tbls. filtered water

Mix all ingredients together, mixture will thicken and soon after it will be necessary to add a little more lemon juice and water to make a spreading consistency like a nut spread. The next day the dip may thicken so a little more liquid may need to be added. This dip is nice served on dark rye sour dough bread or gluten-free crackers.

Tips

Tahini is made from sesame seeds and is a good substitute for dairy as it is full of calcium, and very tasty when the above recipe is used.
No salt is needed in this recipe.
Dark rye sour dough bread can be brought
From good health food stores.

- Best quality tahini can be purchased at Lebanese grocers; ask for imported tahini from Lebanon. ¼ teas. pesto dip can be used as a substitute for chives.

Guacamole Dip

- 1 large ripe avocado (not over –ripe)
- 1 tbls. Spanish onion chopped finely
- 2 tbls. coriander leaves washed and dried well on paper towels
- 1 small bird's eye red chilli, deseeded, chopped finely (optional)
- 1 tbls. lime juice
- Himalayan crystal salt (small aml. ground)
- Ground pepper corns

Mash avocado on large flat plate, chop onion, chilli and coriander finely, separately, then blend all together on a chopping board. Add to avocado with lime juice, salt and pepper. Mix lightly and place in a glass or Pyrex or ceramic dish and refrigerate. Do not cover, but place in an elevated position on top of a bowl with a plate on top of it. This stops the dip from sometimes turning brown, but the taste is not affected. Guacamole is good eaten as a dip or on toast or baked bread or on gluten-free crispbread.

Tips

Dark rye sour dough bread can be brought at good health stores or health cafes. It is best sliced thinly, then placed in freezer in a plastic bag. Take out slices as needed, thaw, then place in an oven set on 175 degrees for several minutes. Cool slightly, then eat with dips or spreads.

Roast Almond Spread

- 250g roasted organic unsalted almonds
- Few drops extra virgin olive oil

Grind almonds in a food processor with attachment, adding olive oil at the beginning of processing. Store in glass jar (not plastic) Makes 1 cup of almond spread.

Tips

- Organic almonds are available at good nut shops. The Champion Juicer has an attachment which grinds all nuts and is easy to operate.

Zucchini Omelette

- 1 egg
- 1 tbls. grated zucchini
- ½ tbls. rice crumbs

- 1 little water
- Salt & Pepper
- 1 tbls. light oil

Whip up egg in dish, add zucchini, crumbs, water and mix well. In a small frying pan heat oil, add egg mixture on low heat, cook for a minute or so, turn and cook for another minute or more until omelette has set. Enjoy.

Variation

- A little sliced and chopped Spanish onion can be added as a variation.
- Add a few shakes of traditional sweet curry powder for a different flavour.

Pan Fried Salmon Or Ocean Trout

- 1 piece salmon or ocean trout(150g) butterflied
- A little light olive oil

Heat oil in a non-stick pot or frying pan, cook fish on low heat for 2 minutes each side and squeeze a little lemon juice, a light twist of salt & pepper and eat with some of the salads set out below.

SALAD

Joe's Coleslaw

- 3 cups white hard cabbage
- 2 cups red cabbage
- 1 large grated carrot, 240grams
- 1 cup finely chopped celery (1 stalk or rib)
- 1½ cups finely chopped flat-leafed parsley
- ¾ cup finely chopped spearmint
- Extra virgin (EV) olive oil and lemon juice

In a large salad bowl (glass or ceramic) 10"x 5" only, not plastic) slice white and red cabbage finely with a sharp knife, and then add carrot, celery parsley and mint in layers. When you want to use it start from the side of the dish as to take even amounts of each vegetable. Take out only what you want to use for that meal. Add olive oil and fresh lemon juice to taste, maybe a little salt and ground pepper corns or cayenne pepper. Replace bowl in refrigerator, covering it with a flat plate (not plastic wrap as food can go off and the taste is affected) Coleslaw should keep for 6-7 days if not used in the next couple of days.

Tips

- The above coleslaw recipe is a large amount saving cutting it up every day. It works best when cut up by hand, not in a food processor as it seems to get over-processed and many vegetable juices are lost, so destroying vitamins and flavour. All vegetables must be fresh including lemon juice.

Beetroot Salad

- 2 cups grated raw beetroot (a large 300g beetroot)
- 4 medium eashallots, or small green onions, washed with tops removed and chopped finely
- ¼ cup chopped flat-leafed parsley finely chopped
- Extra virgin (EV) olive oil
- lemon juicesmall amount ground pepper corns
- no salt needed

Grate beetroot on large grating attachment of food processor. Place in shallow dish or salad plate, add eashallots, parsley and oil and lemon juice. Toss lightly and refrigerate. Cover with a flat plate. Keeps for nearly a week.

Green Salad

- 2 cups baby cos leaves, washed, broken up into bite-sized piece
- ½ stalk celery, sliced finely crossways
- 1 small Lebanese cucumber, sliced finely
- 2 radicchio leaves, washed, cut into bite-sized pieces
- 1 tbls. mint,, finely chopped

- 1 tbls. fennel, sliced finely
- ½ cup EV olive oil
- ¼ cup lemon juice
- Try to omit salt & pepper, as it doesn't need it
  Place all ingredients in a bowl and toss with oil and lemon dressing and serve.

Tips

- Radicchio is an, Italian lettuce, not as soft as other lettuces. It is rather bitter, but is excellent for digestion, containing many anti-oxidants. The above quantity serves 4 persons. If serving less people adjust quantities of salad vegetables and dressing accordingly.
- Lebanese cucumber
- radicchio

Spanish Onion Salad

- 1 large Spanish onion cut in half and sliced finely into half circles
- 1 tbls. mint (not wild) chopped finely
- 1 tbls. EV olive oil
- 1 tbls. lemon juice
- Salt & pepper (optional)

Cut up onion, add mint, oil and lemon and toss well. Place in refrigerator making it about an hour before using it to allow juices to soften the onions and enhance the taste.

Variation

- ½ large thinly sliced fennel can be added to onion and mint to give it more zing.

Joe's Tabouleh

- 3 large bunches continental flat-leaf parsley or to the equivalent of 4 cups finely sliced parsley)
- ¾ cup finely sliced mint
- ¾ cup finely chopped tomatoes (ripe but not over-ripe)
- 4 large eashallots or 4 small ones
- 2 tbls. bur'ghul wheat (optional)
- ½ cup light olive oil
- ¼ cup FRESH lemon juice
- ½ level teas. Lebanese pepper or 5 spices pepper
- Celtic salt & ground pepper corns to taste

Soak bur'ghul in a small bowl by washing and rinsing it with cold water, then drain excess water and leave to stand for ½ hr. until slightly softened.

Next step, cut up UNWASHED parsley finely with a sharp knife on a cutting board. A sharp knife is the best tool. Parsley can be washed at that point in a colander and left to drain for several minutes. It can then be transferred into a large salad bowl and then add all the other ingredients. The last step is to take bur'ghul out of the small bowl, squeeze excess water from it and sprinkle it all over the other ingredients in the salad bowl. Toss tabouleh gently with salad servers to combine flavours of the oil, lemon juice, etc. Refrigerate.

When ready to eat, remove from refrigerator about ten minutes before ready to serve, then toss tabouleh gently with servers to distribute all ingredients and juices evenly.

Tips

It is not recommended to use a food processor to cut any of the above ingredients as a lot of the goodness is lost and will not keep as well.

Using a good sharp knife is the best tool.

- It is not necessary to use bur'ghul for tabouleh. I like to eat tabouleh without bur'ghul these days as it is made from wheat and is better for people with wheat allergies and easier to digest.
- Bur'ghul though can be purchased at Lebanese grocers. Lebanese pepper can also be purchased at Lebanese groceries mostly called "5 spices pepper." Ask for "5 spice pepper" used for tabouleh and Lebanese dishes"

Minestrone

- 2 medium brown onions peeled, cut in half and chopped in small dice
- 2 cloves garlic chopped finely
- 1 large carrot chopped and cut in small dice
- 2 stalks or ribs celery chopped in small dice
- 2 small dark green zucchini cut in small pieces
- 3 cups hard white cabbage sliced medium thickness, about ¼ inch thick
- 5 tbls EV olive oil
- 6 cups filtered water
- ½ cup dried brown lentils or borlotti or romano beans
- 1x400g organic Italian diced tomatoes
- A handful flat-leaf parsley washed and chopped finely
- A few fresh basil leaves broken up (do not cut) or 1 ice cube of pesto (thawed)
- ¼ teas. Himalayan crystal salt
- Ground pepper corns

Always check and remove legumes of grit or stones. Soak beans overnight. Drain water from beans. Place oil in large saucepan and heat oil on low heat, add onions, brown slightly, add garlic and stir, all on low heat, add carrots, celery, zucchini, beans, tomatoes cabbage, basil, rice water salt and pepper. Bring soup to boil on high heat, then lower heat to very low on simmer, stirring regularly to prevent soup from sticking to the saucepan, and adding more water as soup tends to evaporate while cooking. Cook for about 1 ½ hrs to 2hrs or when beans are tender. This soup can be eaten as a main meal or as an entrée. Keeps for about one week in the refrigerator, or can be stored in meal-size plastic containers in freezer to use later on.

Tips

Borlotti or romano beans can be omitted from minestrone but using all other ingredients, and 1 tbsp.raw long grain brown rice can be added, if preferred.

The above quantities of vegetables can be reduced if only wanting to make a small amount of soup, but it is better to make the recipe as written then it can be frozen and stored in the freezer for later use. As with all soups more water than listed may have to be added to saucepan whilst cooking, and stirring regularly to prevent soups from sticking.

Black-Eyed Bean Soup

This under-rated bean is worth trying.

- 1 ½ cups dried black-eyed beans
- 1 large onion, chopped finely
- 2 plump cloves garlic, chopped finely

- 2 tbls. fresh dill leaves chopped finely
- 1 handful flat leaf parsley, chopped finely
- 1 large outer stalk or rib of celery, chopped finely
- ¼ teas. Himalayan crystal salt
- 4 tbls. fresh lemon juice
- 5 tbls. EV cold-pressed olive oil
- About 5-6 cups litre filtered water
- Extra water

Soak beans overnight. Drain water and wash beans well and check for any dirt or grit. In a large saucepan brown onion on low heat, add garlic and cook for a minute, and whilst still on low heat, add celery, black-beans beans, parsley, dill leaves and salt and pepper corns and water. Place lid on saucepan, bring to boil on high heat, then lower heat down to a simmer, adding more water as necessary (about 4 extra cups) as soup tends to evaporate, and stir regularly to avoid soup from sticking to saucepan. Cook for about 2 hrs or less depending on tenderness of beans or when beans are cooked to the desired consistency. This soup can be eaten as is or I prefer to eat it half or slightly blitzed as it more hearty and seems to have more taste and bulk and fibre. This soup can be eaten freshly cooked or some of it stored in freezer for later use. Soups keep for several months in freezer.

Dahl Or Red Lentil Soup

- 2 cups red lentils (checked and washed for grit and stones)
- 1 large brown onion, cut into small dice
- 2 cloves garlic, finely chopped
- 1 flat tbls. fresh ginger root, peeled and finely chopped or grated
- 2 level teas. ground cumin
- 12 Curry leaves
- Few shakes chilli powder or (½ small red birds eye chilli) may be hot (optional)
- Few shakes cayenne pepper
- About 5-6cups filtered water
- ¼ teas. Himalayan crystal salt
- Ground pepper corns
- 5 tbls. EV olive oil

Heat oil in large saucepan. Add onion and cook until soft for approx. 2 minutes. Add garlic, ginger and cook for 1 minute. Season to taste with salt and pepper. Add turmeric, cumin, cayenne and chilli powder and heat through for 2 minutes stirring constantly on low heat. Add washed and drained red lentils and stir to coat with spices. Bring to the boil, reduce heat to simmer, stirring regularly, with lid partially covered for about 40 minutes or when mixture is a thick soupy consistency, almost pureed. Whilst stirring regularly, it may be necessary to add extra water to this soup as it has a tendency to adhere to the saucepan. There is no need to puree this soup as it is good to eat as is. When cooled, pour into bowls and refrigerate.

Tips

- This soup tastes better the next day after it is cooked as food cooked with spices settle and flavour is improved. This mixture is a large amount so when cooled some can be stored in the refrigerator in containers for later use.

Brussell Sprout Minestrone

Brussell sprouts never tasted like these.

- 6 medium-sized brussell sprouts, (tops removed and cut in quarters)
- 1 leek (whites only, cut in half and washed well)
- 1 medium brown onion, peeled, cut in half and cut into small dice
- 2 cloves garlic, peeled and chopped finely
- 1 medium carrot, peeled and cut into small dice
- 1 stalk or rib celery, outside skin peeled and cut up small
- 1 small dark green zucchini, chopped small
- 8 fresh basil leaves, uncut
- 1 x 400g can organic Italian diced tomatoes
- 1 tbs of uncooked Brown rice
- ¼ teas. Himalayan crystal salt
- Ground pepper corns
- A handful of finely chopped flat-leaf parsley

- 5 tbls. EV olive oil
- About 5 cups filtered water

Place oil in a large saucepan and heat oil gently on low heat. Wash vegetables well. Add onion leek, still on low heat saute for a couple of minutes until soft, then add garlic, carrot, celery, zucchini, tomatoes, parsley, basil leaves, rice and salt and peppercorns and water. Cover vegetables with water with lid on, bringing to boil on high heat, then continue cooking on a very low heat, stirring regularly so mixture doesn't stick to the saucepan or burn. More water will have to be added to the pot while cooking. Cook for about 1 hr. or less, when sprouts are tender when tested with a skewer and it comes out easily. Cool, pour into bowls and refrigerate. Can be frozen for later use.

Tips

- 3 cups firmly packed of hard white cabbage (sliced finely) can be substituted for brussell sprouts. This soup can be eaten as an entrée or perhaps as a complete meal, or as a side-dish.
- If fresh basil is not available a frozen cube of pesto can be used.

(recipe below)

Celeriac Soup

- 1 celeriac, about 750g, peeled, cut into 2 inch. or 5 cm. pieces
- 1 medium size potato, peeled and cut in 4 pieces
- 1 large leek, whites only, cut in half longways and washed well, cut into thin slices
- 1 medium size onion, peeled and cut in half and into small dice
- 2 large cloves garlic, chopped
- 1 ½ inch piece fresh ginger root, grated or chopped finely
- 2 tbls. fresh dill leaves, chopped finely
- 5-6 cups filtered water
- ¼ teas. Himalayan crystal salt
- Ground pepper corns
- 4 tbls. EV olive oil

Wash ingredients well. Heat oil, brown onion until softened, add garlic, then rest of ingredients. Cook for about half and hour or until celeriac is cooked. Test with skewer.

Tips

Celeriac is a knobbly, gnarly root vegetable available during winter months.
- Although celeriac is a starchy vegetable, it contains less starch than other root vegetables

- like potatoes, pumpkin or parsnips, making it an ideal low-starch, tasty and healthy soup.
- Celeriac can also be cut in chunks like baked potatoes, placed on baking paper, with a drizzle of oil, and a dash of cayenne pepper, cooking for half and hour, then turning pieces over and cooked for another half hour.

Cauliflower Soup

- 1x750g whole cauliflower,
- 1 large brown onion, cut in half and small dice
- 1 large leek, trimmed, cut longways and cut into thin slices
- 2 medium cloves garlic, chopped finely
- 2 heaped. tbls. chopped coriander and some stalks
- 1½ inch. piece ginger, chopped finely
- 1 ½ teas. cumin powder
- Few shakes chilli powder
- Few shakes cayenne pepper
- Ground pepper corns
- ¼ teas. Himalayan crystal salt
- 4 tbls. EV olive oil
- 5-6 cups filtered water

Cut outside leaves from cauliflower, the small young leaves can be left on. Cut up cauliflower into medium sized florets. Heat oil in large saucepan on low heat, add onions, leek, cook for a few minutes, add garlic, ginger, cauliflower, 1 cup of water, coriander, and spices, stirring and coating cauliflower with spices for a couple of minutes, then add rest of water. Bring to boil on high heat, lower heat to simmer and cook for about 30-40 minutes until cauliflower is tender, stirring regularly, adding more water if necessary. You can tell when it is cooked, when tested with a skewer and it comes out easily. Cool slightly, process with stick blender to desired consistency, semi-bulky or fine. I prefer to eat it with a bit of bulk and body. Pour into bowls and refrigerate.

Tips

Variation
Spices can be substituted for 2 tbls. chopped dill leaves for the above soup.

A medium-size potato may be added

Lamb Chop Casserole With Rosemary, Garlic And Red Wine

- 4-6 lamb chump chops
- 1 large brown onion, cut in half and into small dice
- 1 tbls. fresh rosemary, sliding stems from stalk with hands and cut up finely
- 2 medium cloves garlic
- 2 tbls. rice flour
- 2 tbls. EV cold pressed olive oil
- ½ cup red wine
- 2 cups or more of filtered water to start

- ¼ teas. Himalayan crystal salt
- Ground pepper corns

Trim chops of excess fat. Place chops and rice flour and salt in a plastic bag and toss. Heat oil in large, non-stick frying pan, fry chops for about 2 minutes or more until brown and turn over for another two minutes. Remove chops and place on absorbent paper or paper towels. Add a bit more oil and fry onions and garlic until soft, a couple of minutes, add rosemary and wine and stir on low heat for another couple of minutes. Replace chops in pan and add water and cover with lid. Bring to boil on high heat, then lower to simmer, stirring regularly to prevent chops from sticking and adding more water as casserole evaporates. Cook for 1 ½ -2 hrs. depending on tenderness of meat. Test with skewer; it is cooked when skewer inserted into chops comes out easily.

Tips

- Chops can be substituted with blade or stewing steak which work well, but I like to cook casseroles using chops, rather than boneless meat, and chicken on the bone as well, as they always seem to have more flavour. I guess it is a personal choice. This casserole can be cooked in the oven, sealed with foil, but it will have to be checked regularly, maybe adding more water and basting and to prevent from sticking.

Veal Chops Cacciatore

- 4 veal rib eye chops
- Few fresh sage leaves
- 1 teas. dried sage leaves
- 2 medium cloves garlic
- A handful flat-leafed parsley, chopped finely, leaves only
- ½ cup white wine (any)
- 1 x 400g Italian organic diced tomatoes
- 2 tbls. EV cold pressed olive oil
- ¼ teas. of Himalayan crystal salt
- 8 whole peppercorns
- Filtered water

Heat oil in non-stick frypan, add chops and brown for a few minutes each side. Add garlic, sage and parsley and wine on low heat and stir for a few minutes to combine. Add salt and peppercorns and tomatoes. Bring to the boil on high heat, lower heat down to simmer, adding more water if necessary, keeping an eye so veal doesn't stick to pan. Cover with lid and cook for about 1 ½ hrs. or more until meat is tender. Alternatively this casserole can be cooked in the oven covered with foil for the same time, basting and adding more water, if necessary.

Baked Garlic And Lemon Chicken

- 4-6 medium size thigh cutlets with skin on, (on bone) also known as chicken chops
- ¼ cup EV cold-pressed olive oil
- ¼ cup FRESH lemon juice
- 4 large cloves garlic, chopped finely
- Himalayan Salt & pepper corns

In a corning ware or ceramic dish place lemon juice, oil and peeled chopped garlic, and then chicken pieces. Score chicken on skin side, making slight slits in 3 places. Stir chicken and juices well together, add salt and pepper. Bake in a moderate oven, fan-forced about 175o uncovered for about 40 minutes, basting with juices. Turn chicken over and baste and cook for another 30 minutes or less until browned. You know they are cooked when a skewer inserted comes out easily. Cooking times varies with different ovens.

Tips

- This recipe can be cooked using other chicken pieces. Thigh cutlets can be substituted for a whole chicken, a size 15 which your butcher can cut into 8 pieces leaving extra flesh on the wing bone. Other pieces that can be used are ½ breasts on the bone, or chicken drumsticks. Boneless chicken does not work as well for this recipe.

Extra lemon juice and oil may have to be added for any extra pieces cooked.

Salmon With Rosemary, Garlic And Lemon Zest

- 2 fillets fresh salmon, 150g each, butterflied
- 1 tbls. fresh rosemary, chopped finely
- 2 medium cloves garlic, chopped finely
- ½ tbls. rice flour
- Zest and a dash of fresh lemon juice
- Few grains of Himalayan salt
- Ground peppercorns
- 1 tbls. EV olive oil
- ¾ - 1 cup filtered water

Prepare all ingredients first. Firstly remove the thin outer layer of brown skin of salmon with a sharp knife. Butterfly cut each piece of salmon. Grate lemon zest, slide rosemary leaves from stem and cut up very finely and add along with lemon zest into a small bowl. In another bowl dissolve rice flour in water and combine. Heat oil in small non-stick, frying pan. On low heat fry fish for 2 minutes on one side, turn over and cook for 1 minute. Remove from heat and let it rest for one minute. Add lemon zest mixture and stir for another minute with a non-stick spoon. Replace pan on stove, then add flour dissolved in water with lemon juice. Stir gently to coat mixture on fish. Cook on low heat for about 5 minutes or until a skewer inserted comes out easily. Serve with mashed or baked carrots or swede and green leafy vegetables.

Tips

- Fresh salmon can be bought in bulk amounts (1 kilo) for convenience. Cut up salmon in chunks or fillets of 150g each. Wrap individually in plastic wrap to store in freezer and use when needed.

Sweet Curried Borlotti Bean Casserole

- 2 cups borlotti or romano dried beans
- 1 large brown onion, chopped in small dice
- 1 large granny smith apple, peeled, cut in half and cut into small dice
- 2 cloves garlic, peeled and chopped finely
- 2 tbls. fresh lemon juice
- 5 tbls. EV cold-pressed olive oil
- 1 level teas. traditional sweet curry powder (I like Keens brand)
- 1 level teas. turmeric powder
- ¼ teas. Himalayan crystal salt
- Ground pepper corns
- 5 cups filtered water

Place beans on paper and look carefully to remove any grit or stones as they can cause serious dental problems if a tooth is inadvertently cracked whilst eating them. (as with all legumes) Then soak beans overnight in enough water to cover. Next day drain water off and rinse clean. In a large saucepan heat oil, then add onion and apple, stirring and cook until lightly browned on low heat. Add beans and curry and turmeric, still on low heat, stirring to coat beans with spices for a few minutes. Add lemon juice, salt and pepper and water. Cover with lid and bring to boil on high heat, lower to simmer, stirring regularly and adding more water as bean stew evaporates. Cook for 1 ½ -2 hrs depending on desired tenderness. Cool on stove and pour into bowls and refrigerate. Can be frozen and keeps for several months in freezer. The above dish is good eaten with a rice pilaf.

Tips

- This dish tastes better the next day after it is made, but does not work as well using canned beans, as salt content is high and the texture is not the same. It is better to do the extra work and enjoy the flavour of the dried beans. Borlotti or romano beans can be substituted for chops or blade or chuck steak. Lamb neck or lamb chump chops work well with the above recipe.

Spaghetti Ragout With Italian Pork And Fennel Sausage

- 6 thin Italian pork and fennel sausages (each sausage cut into 4 pieces)
- 6x400g organic Italian diced tomatoes, pureed with hand blender)
- ½ cup red wine (good quality)
- 2 large onions, cut in halves, cut into small dice
- 6 large cloves garlic, peeled and cut finely
- Handful fresh basil leaves, uncut
- ½ flat tbls refined celtic sea salt
- Ground pepper corns
- 4 tbls. EV cold-pressed olive oil

In a large non-stick casserole saucepan heat 1 tbl. oil, add sausages and cook for a few minutes caramelising slightly until lightly browned, add onion, cook slightly, add garlic, then wine and cook for several minutes stirring lightly. Puree tomatoes, in a separate bowl, add basil leaves, salt & peppercorns. Cook for about 1 to 1 ¼ hrs or longer, or when sauce has thickened. No extra water is needed for cooking sauce. The above quantity of spaghetti ragout is a large quantity. I prefer to make it in bulk and store in plastic containers, adding the same amount of sausage pieces to each container. Keeps for several months but should not be stored for an extended time.

Tips

One large pork chop, cut in half and a thick slice chuck steak cut up in chunks can be substituted for Italian sausages.

- As a variation olives, and or anchovies can also be added to the above sauce for extra flavour, but I prefer to eat the above sauce as is because of the high salt content of salty additives. It already has enough flavour. I do not use tomato paste for the same reason. My choice of spaghetti is Orgran or Buon Tempo Brand, and my favourite shapes are Spaghetti No. 5 and Buon Tempo gluten and wheat-free spirals or penne.

Pesto For Pasta Or Rice

- 3 cups fresh basil leaves, washed and stalks removed, firmly packed
- 3 plump cloves garlic
- ¼ teas. Himalayan sea salt
- 1/3 cup extra virgin olive oil
- ¼ cup pine nuts, toasted
- 1 tbls. pecorino cheese, or more to taste grated (optional)

In a stick blended bowl or food processor place basil leaves, chopped garlic, salt and olive oil. Process for several seconds, remove lid and scrape sides of bowl, replace lid, add pinenuts that have been lightly toasted and process further until pesto is rather smooth. Extra oil may have to be added, a bit at a time to loosen and make it smooth and prevent it from discolouring. Cheese should not be added to pesto until ready to serve with pasta. This recipe yields 6 tbls. pesto. Can be stored in freezer for later use.

Tips

- 250g pasta usually needs about 3 tbls. pesto. Cheese can be omitted for those who choose not to eat dairy or those who are lactose intolerant. Cheese should not be added to pesto if freezing it as it does not freeze well. Alternatively, fresh left-over pesto can be stored in ice cube trays in the freezer for single use, as in Pesto with minestrone recipe, Brussell sprout minestrone, or cabbage recipe with pesto, (recipe below)

LEBANESE RECIPE SECTION

The recipes below have been inspired by three trail-blazer Lebanese sisters who co-wrote the FIRST Lebanese Cookbook in Australia. It is entitled "Lebanese Cookbook" by sisters, Dawn, Elaine and Selwa Anthony, and it was first published in Australia in 1978.

Kibbi

- 1½ lbs. small lean shoulder of lamb (boned and minced finely, not coarse)
- 1½ cups bur'ghul , washed and rinsed off water
- 2 large brown onions, peeled, cut in half and cut up rather smallish
- 1 medium bird's eye chilli, cut finely
- ½ teas. Lebanese pepper
- 2 tbls. celtic sea salt, fine
- 1 cup light olive oil

Wash bur'ghul in large bowl and rinse off water. Let stand for an hour before mixing in food processor. Heat oven at 220o. While oven is heating, cut up ingredients. Bur'ghul will swell and rise, add a little water on top of it. Mix well with other ingredients by dividing into two batches to go into food prcedssor, mix half of minced lamb, half of onions and half of chilli and half of bur'ghul, half of chilli, half of bur'ghul, half of salt and pepper and place in food processor and mix for several seconds, turn off processor and scrape sides of bowl once or twice. Process until well combined and remove from processor and turn onto a plate. Process second batch the same way. Mix both batches together with hands and then place into a well-oiled baking tray measuring about 15x10 ½ x 1 ½. Wet hands with a little water, making it easier to spread,, and flatten meat mixture evenly in tray. Pour oil evenly all over kibbi mixture, then cut diagonal shapes right through the meat to allow oil to penetrate. Tilt tray slightly so oil can spread to all sides of the tray. Bake kibbi on centre shelf of oven on high heat for 20 mins then transfer to the top shelf of oven and cook for about another ½ hr. Slices from the side cook quicker than the centre slices, so keep an eye on them, and removed when they are nicely browned. Centre slices take a little longer Remove slices with a v-shaped trowel, making careful slices don't stick to tray. Meat is cooked when slices are browned, not burned, and slide out evenly, with care. All of the kibbi should be cooked in under an hour. Remove slices as they are cooked and place on flat platter on absorbent paper towels. Cool well and refrigerate. When cold cover with foil. Can be eaten with salads and as an accompaniment to other Lebanese dishes. Delish!

Hoummus B'tahini

- 1 ½ cups dried chick peas
- 3-4 tbls. tahini
- ¼ cup lemon juice
- 4 large cloves garlic, peeled and chopped smallish
- 2 tbls. reserved water from chick peas (keep in jar)
- Olive oil and sweet paprika to garnish
- 1 flat teas. fine celtic sea salt (to taste)

Soak peas overnight in water in large bowl. Next day rinse off water and place in saucepan with filtered water to cover. Bring to boil and cook on low heat for ¾ -1hr. depending on tenderness. More water will have to be added during cooking as peas evaporate and can stick to saucepan or burn. Keep an eye on them and stir. To test squash onto a spoon with another spoon and when they are soft, they are cooked. Drain and reserve half of the water and cool. When cool place peas in food processor, add garlic, lemon juice, tahini and 2 tbls reserved water. Process for a few seconds, turn off processor and scrape mixture from sides of bowl and continue processing until mixture is at the desired consistency. I like the hummus to have a bit of texture to it or it can be mixed finer. Pour into a bowl and refrigerate. The next day the hummus will thicken up in the fridge; more liquids will need to be added, a little more reserved water, maybe a little lemon and maybe a little salt to taste. Place hummus on flat platter, spreading evenly and decorate with a light drizzle of EV olive oil and finely sprinkled sweet paprika. Serve with bar-b-qued meats, kibbi, chicken, etc.

TIPS

Canned beans don't work well in the above recipe; the texture is softer and flavour is not as good as the dried variety, also the canned variety contain more salt.

This dish is well worth starting from scratch using dried beans for the flavour and texture is worth the extra effort, plus the health benefits.

Green Beans In Oil

- 800g. stringless beans
- 1/3 cup EV cold pressed olive oil
- 2 large brown onions, peeled, cut in half, in small dice
- ½ teas. black pepper
- 1 teas. fine celtic sea salt
- 1-1½ cups filtered water

Top and tail beans and then cut beans in half. Heat the oil in large saucepan and fry the onions until they are reddish-brown. Mix in the beans, salt and pepper. Saute for 10 minutes on low heat. Stir in about ¾ cup water at first, cover and simmer very slowly, adding more water if necessary until the beans are almost soft. Remove lid and continue cooking uncovered to absorb excess juice. When cooked the beans should be very brown and consistency according to taste, either a bit chewy or soft. Serve eaten with Lebanese bread, or as an accompaniment to Lebanese dishes or bar-b-ques etc.

TIPS

Lebanese beans are delicious eaten for breakfast. First get a slice of dark rye sourdough bread (plain or lightly baked) and spread on some tahini dip and then a large spoonful of beans on top.

Garlic Sauce Or Dip

- 1 large whole head or corm of garlic, heads separated, peeled, and ends removed (do not cut)
- 1 level teas. fine celtic sea salt
- 2 cups light olive oil
- Approx. ¼ cup fresh lemon juice

This is a tricky dish to make successfully. The authors recommend to crush the garlic with a mortar and pestle until the salt is dissolved. I like to make it in a food processor. Place garlic in food processor, mix, after about ten seconds start to gradually add oil, a few drops at a time, continue beating, gradually adding more oil, continue beating until mixture becomes fluffy. Very gradually start to add lemon juice (a few drops at a time) beat for a while, and then gradually adding more oil alternately with rest of lemon juice, until all liquids have been added. Continue beating until mixture resembles a meringue with peaks or fluffy like mashed potato. Garlic sauce should resemble mashed potato but with more density.

Tips

Garlic sauce is delicious eaten with bar-b-qued meats, chicken, fish, etc.

- This dish requires practice and if at the start the mixture falls flat, it is useless to continue, maybe just stop there and then, don't waste any more oil. Don't throw mixture out, it can be used in the cooking for flavouring foods. Refrigerate. When making garlic sauce it is also important to use a strong, efficient food processor with blades that are situated in the right place and reach the sides of the bowl.
- If the above recipe proves too difficult to made, there are packaged Garlic Sauces which taste just as good as restaurant quality. These can be purchased at lebanese grocers or supermarkets.
- Monjay Brand is a good one.

Mushroom, Spinach and Pesto Risotto

- 2 medium b. onions, diced
- 2-3 cloves garlic, crushed or chopped finely
- 200g baby spinach leaves, approx.
- 1½ cups half-cooked brown long grain rice
- 1 large Portobello mushroom, approx 300g, finely sliced
- ½ cup white wine
- 3 tbls. EV olive oil
- 1½ tbls. pesto
- 4-6 cups water
- Himalayan salt & ground pepper corns
- 2 tbls. pecorino cheese, grated (optional)

Heat 2 tbls. oil in a frying pan over medium-high heat. Stir in the mushrooms and cook until soft for about 3 minutes. Remove mushrooms and their liquid from the pan and set aside.

Heat 1 tbls. remaining oil in pan, on medium heat, add onions first, cook until soft, add garlic, stirring to prevent from sticking. Add rice, stirring to coat with oil, add water, wine, salt and pepper, stirring constantly until the wine and water is fully absorbed. Cook until the rice is al dente or to preferred consistency, about 15mins. Add mushrooms, pesto, cheese and spinach leaves and stir well to combine.

Tips

How to half cook brown long grain rice. Rice can be cooked in bulk rather than 1½ cup lots at a time. I like to cook 3-4 cups raw long grain brown rice beforehand, (the day before is best). Place rice which has been rinsed with filtered water into a large non-stick saucepan and add about 2 cups filtered water. Cover and bring to the boil on high heat; remove lid and simmer on low heat for fifteen minutes, adding more cold water as necessary as rice dries up. Drain, rinse off water and pour into a metal colander (not a plastic colander as plastic will make the rice swell and over-cook) The rice is now half-cooked. Cool well until rice is quite cold, then place 1½ cup lots of rice in plastic containers and freeze for later use.

Cabbage With Pesto Sauce

- 4 cups hard white cabbage, sliced, ¼ inch. thick
- 1 medium brown onion, cut in half, in small dice
- 1 flat tbls. pesto sauce
- ground pepper (If needed)
- 2 tbls. EV olive oil
- ½ cup water

Heat oil in large non-stick frying pan, add onion and brown slightly, on low heat. Add pesto and stir, add water to prevent from sticking, then add cabbage and stir. Place lid on cabbage and cook for about 5 minutes. Serve as a side dish to meat and chicken, dishes, etc.

Tips

- Red cabbage can be substituted for white cabbage, which is richer in anti-oxidants than white.
- Savoy cabbage does not work for this dish as it is too soft.

RED CABBAGE GERMAN STYLE

This recipe is another variation of a red cabbage dish, also a healthy vegetarian option.

1 lb. red cabbage, sliced about ¼ inch thick
4 tbls. Ev olive oil
 1 large diced b. onion
1 cup of filtered water
½ small green apple, peeled and sliced
pinch of nutmeg
1 pinch ground cinnamon
Salt and ground pepper to taste

Heat oil in large non-stick frying pan or pot over medium heat; add onions, stirring until lightly browned and translucent, about 6 to 8 minutes. Stir in water, apple slices and bring to boil. Stir in nutmeg, cinnamon, salt and pepper. Stir in red cabbage, cover, bring to boil and reduce heat to a low simmer, stirring occasionally, until cabbage is soft and cooked through, 30-45 mins or less according to taste.

Tips

The above dish is a delicious side dish eaten with a protein dish, fish or any starch meal.

Sauteed Chicory

This recipe is inspired by Miraglia Eriquez and a high-fibre dish.

- 1 bunch chicory, about 500g)
- 3 -4 tbls. extra virgin olive oil
- 3 cloves garlic, peeled and chopped finely
- 1 small bird's eye chilli, chopped and deseeded
- ¼ teas. Himalayan sea salt
- Ground pepper corns

Cut stalks from chicory. Cut into 3 inch intervals and wash well in cold water. Drain in colander. Place in saucepan and cover generously with filtered water. Bring to boil and cook for 10-15 minutes until almost tender. Drain in colander. You can reserve the water for drinking later on. Cool chicory slightly, then heat oil in large non-stick frying pan, add garlic and chilli, stir on low heat until nearly brown, then add chicory and a tbls. reserved water, stirring continually. Cover with lid and cook for another 5 or 10 minutes or until it reaches the desired tenderness.

Tips

- Chicory is a long-leaf rather bitter green vegetable available all the year round, but it tastes best in the winter months. It is available in summer months and it can be a little strong, however we eat it all year long. Although it is a slightly bitter-tasting vegetable, it is worth trying, if it is dressed-up, as above, or in a soup or stew. It is a good idea to keep the water chicory is cooked in and drink it warmed as it is a good blood-cleanser and excellent for digestion.

The above dish can be eaten as a side dish or along with other vegetables for a vegetarian option or if trying to lose weight.